YOUR COMPLETE VEGAN
Pregnancy

Your All-in-One Guide to a Healthy, Holistic, Plant-Based Pregnancy

REED MANGELS, PhD, RD

Adams Media
New York   London   Toronto   Sydney   New Delhi

Adams**media**

Adams Media
An Imprint of Simon & Schuster, Inc.
57 Littlefield Street
Avon, Massachusetts 02322

First Adams Media trade paperback edition April 2019

ADAMS MEDIA and colophon are trademarks of Simon & Schuster.

For information about special discounts for bulk purchases, please contact Simon & Schuster Special Sales at 1-866-506-1949 or business@simonandschuster.com.

The Simon & Schuster Speakers Bureau can bring authors to your live event. For more information or to book an event contact the Simon & Schuster Speakers Bureau at 1-866-248-3049 or visit our website at www.simonspeakers.com.

Interior design by Heather McKiel
Interior images © Getty Images

Manufactured in the United States of America

10 9 8 7 6 5 4 3 2

Library of Congress Cataloging-in-Publication Data
Names: Mangels, Reed, author.
Title: Your complete vegan pregnancy / Reed Mangels, PhD, RD.
Description: Avon, Massachusetts: Adams Media, 2019.
Includes bibliographical references and index.
Identifiers: LCCN 2018055401 | ISBN 9781507210192 (pb) | ISBN 9781507210208 (ebook)
Subjects: LCSH: Pregnancy--Health aspects. | Pregnancy--Nutritional aspects. | Childbirth. | Veganism. | Vegan cooking.
Classification: LCC RG559 .M344 2019 | DDC 618.2/42--dc23
LC record available at https://lccn.loc.gov/2018055401

ISBN 978-1-5072-1019-2
ISBN 978-1-5072-1020-8 (ebook)

Contains material adapted from the following title published by Adams Media, an Imprint of Simon & Schuster, Inc.: *The Everything® Vegan Pregnancy Book* by Reed Mangels, PhD, RD, LD, FADA, copyright © 2011, ISBN 978-1-4405-2551-3.

Contents

The Basics

Chapter 1

Vegan Diets: The Basics

Whether you've been vegan for many years, are a relative newcomer to veganism, or are simply contemplating being vegan, adding pregnancy to the equation may raise some questions for you. Rest assured, the Academy of Nutrition and Dietetics (formerly the American Dietetic Association) has said that well-planned vegan diets are "appropriate for all stages of the life cycle, including pregnancy…[and] lactation."

Pregnancy (or prepregnancy) is a great time to learn more about vegan nutrition so that you can be sure you are making the best possible food choices!

Vegan Defined

The Vegan Society, which was formed in 1944 and is based in the United Kingdom, defines *veganism* as "a way of living which seeks to exclude, as far as is possible and practicable, all forms of exploitation of, and cruelty to, animals for food, clothing or any other purpose." The Vegetarian Resource Group, a nonprofit educational group in the United States, states, "Vegetarians do not eat meat, fish, or poultry. Vegans, in addition to being vegetarian, do not use other animal products and by-products such as eggs, dairy products, honey, leather, fur, silk, wool, cosmetics, and soaps derived from animal products."

To simplify, vegans avoid using animal products and foods or ingredients derived from animal products. Some ingredients derived from animal products may be fairly obvious, such as chicken or beef broth or casein from milk. Other ingredients may be less apparent, though. Gelatin, for example, is derived from animal bones and connective tissue. Carmine (sometimes called *cochineal*) is a red food coloring derived from the dried bodies of female beetles. These are examples of ingredients that vegans avoid. Whether you've been vegan for years or just started, you are probably already very familiar with reading ingredient listings on products and making decisions about which products or ingredients fit into your values scheme.

Strangely enough, there are no federal rules regulating the use of *vegan* on labels of products. Some private companies and nonprofit organizations have developed their own standards and guidelines as to what a vegan food is. That's why it is always recommended that to determine if a food meets your definition of vegan, check the ingredient listing!

Vegans also try to avoid foods that may have used animal products in their production. For example, some sugar companies process sugar through a bone char in order to remove color from the sugar. Wine production may also involve animal products. Clarifying agents for wine include egg whites, casein (from milk), gelatin, and isinglass (from fish). Foods fortified with vitamin D contain one of two forms of vitamin D: either D_2 or D_3. Vitamin D_3 is typically made from lanolin, an oily substance from sheep's wool.

What Are Vegan Foods?

Vegans eat a wide variety of foods, many of which are familiar to those eating a more traditional American diet. For example, a vegan breakfast could include orange juice, toast with jelly, oatmeal with raisins, and coffee or tea. Lunch could be a standard PB and J sandwich with an apple and some chips, while dinner could be bean burritos, a tossed salad with Italian dressing, and apple crisp.

Vegans may also choose some foods that can seem less familiar. For instance, breakfast could include vegan "sausage" and pancakes, lunch could feature a veggie burger, and dinner could be barbecued seitan (pronounced *say-tan*) over quinoa with vegan biscuits and a frozen dessert based on coconut milk.

Many foods traditionally made with animal products are available in vegan form in large supermarkets and natural foods stores. From macaroni and cheese to fish sticks to barbecue ribs, there are many convenient (and delicious) vegan options available.

In addition, vegan cookbooks and websites offer recipes for making vegan versions of nonvegan foods. Recipes may include simple tricks like replacing eggs with flaxseed or tofu, or they may feature more complicated formulas to make dishes that taste like seafood or dairy-based cheese.

And nowadays, many restaurants have vegan options on their menus as well. If you don't see something that you like, don't hesitate to ask if there are vegan versions available. Chefs are often happy to create a dish that meets your dietary needs. Ethnic restaurants frequently have vegan dishes or dishes that could easily be made vegan. Here are a few ideas:

- Veggie no-cheese pizza—make sure to get lots of your favorite vegetable toppings. Ask if the dough contains cheese, milk, or eggs.
- Moo shu vegetables—ask your server to tell the kitchen to leave out eggs.
- Falafel—crunchy chickpea balls in a pita pocket with a spicy sauce.
- Indian curries and dal—ask to be made with oil instead of ghee (clarified butter).
- Bean burritos and tacos—hold the cheese and sour cream; check for lard in refried beans.
- Pasta with mushroom or marinara sauce (hold the Parmesan).
- Ethiopian injera and lentil stew.

Fitting a Vegan Diet to Your Lifestyle

When you decide to become vegan, there are no specific requirements as to how much (or how little) cooking you will need to do. Some vegans love to prepare meals and create new recipes. They may have shelves of cookbooks and the latest cooking equipment, while other vegans rely on takeout, convenience foods, and quick-to-fix meals. You may find yourself at one of these extremes or somewhere in the middle. You may even vary your style from day to day. It's important to remember that you absolutely can make a vegan diet fit your food and cooking preferences. If you want to be a foodie, there are plenty of opportunities to try new ingredients and seek out new techniques. If you need to make dinner in twenty minutes, convenience foods like canned beans, precut vegetables, and quick-cooking pasta are just what you need.

According to a 2016 poll commissioned in the United States by The Vegetarian Resource Group, approximately 1.5 percent of the adult population consistently follows a vegan diet. This is up from 1 percent in 2009. That means approximately 3.7 million adults in the United States are vegan. There are 4.3 million adult vegetarians in the US, about half of which is female and half is male.

Key Nutrients You Need

The key to a nutritionally sound vegan diet is actually quite simple. Eating a variety of foods, including fruits, vegetables, plenty of leafy greens, whole-grain products, beans, nuts, and seeds, virtually ensures that you'll meet most of your nutrient needs. Subsequent chapters will provide additional details about specific nutrients that are important to be aware of.

There is one nutrient in particular that vegans are asked about most often: protein. Although many foods provide some protein, the dried bean family is an especially good way to get protein when you are following a vegan diet. From vegetarian baked beans to chili *sin carne* (without meat) to lentil soup, it's easy to add beans to your diet. Soy products such as tofu, tempeh, soy milk, textured vegetable protein (TVP), and edamame are also high in protein. And don't forget whole grains, nuts, nut butters, vegetables, potatoes, and seeds (pumpkin, sesame, sunflower, etc.) that are also great ways to add to your protein totals.

When you are following a vegan diet, your iron and zinc needs increase because these are not absorbed as easily from beans and grains. There are some tricks to increase your absorption of these minerals. Including a food with vitamin C (citrus, tomatoes, cabbage, or broccoli, for instance) at most meals can markedly boost iron and zinc absorption. Good sources of iron and zinc for vegans include enriched breakfast cereals, wheat germ, soy products, dried beans, pumpkin and sunflower seeds, and dark chocolate.

On a per-calorie basis, many of the top iron sources are vegan. For instance, a 100-calorie portion of cooked spinach supplies almost 16 milligrams of iron, and 100 calories of Swiss chard provides over 11 milligrams. Compare that to 100 calories of broiled sirloin steak supplying less than a milligram of iron or to 100 calories of skim milk with one-tenth of a milligram of iron.

Calcium and vitamin D are key for strong bones, so it's important to make sure you are getting enough from your diet. Some vegan foods are fortified with calcium and vitamin D. Check labels of soy milk and other plant milks to make sure they have calcium and vitamin D added to them. Calcium is also found in foods like dark leafy greens, tofu set with calcium salts, and dried figs. Vitamin D can also be produced by your skin when you're out in the sun. Vegan vitamin D supplements are another way to meet your vitamin D needs. And, of course, exercise is a key requirement for building strong bones as well, so don't skip out on breaking a sweat!

Vitamin B_{12} cannot be reliably obtained from unfortified vegan foods, but there are vegan foods that are fortified with this important vitamin. Fortified foods include some brands of breakfast cereals, nutritional yeast, plant-based milks, and mock meats. If you're not sure whether or not you're getting enough vitamin B_{12} from fortified foods, a vitamin B_{12} supplement is a wise idea.

Fish and fish oils are often promoted as sources of omega-3 fatty acids. Vegans have other options. You can get omega-3s from flaxseeds, flax oil, walnuts, hemp seeds, and other foods. There are even vegan versions of the omega-3 fatty acids found in fish oil—DHA and EPA.

According to a 2016 position paper on vegetarian diets by the Academy of Nutrition and Dietetics, by making smart food choices, it's easy to eat a healthy vegan diet—one that's good for you, for your baby-to-be, and for the planet.

Why Choose Veganism?

People choose to be vegan for many different reasons. Some people initially become vegan for health reasons—perhaps they've had a health crisis or want to reduce the risk of their family history of heart disease or cancer. Other people choose not to use any animal products because they know that there are alternatives that do not involve hurting animals. A person's reasons for being vegan may evolve over time also. For example, someone who originally became vegan due to concerns about animals notices significant health benefits from a vegan diet. Someone who became vegan following a heart attack may go on to read more about factory farms and continue to be vegan to help animals as well.

> Every year, over nine million chickens and turkeys are slaughtered in the United States. And more than one hundred million cattle, pigs, and sheep are killed annually.

For the Animals

Some people choose to be vegan because they believe that eating eggs and dairy products promotes the meat industry. For example, male chickens not needed for egg production are killed. Male calves are often raised for veal production. And when cows or egg-laying chickens are no longer productive, they are often sold for meat.

Add these issues to others, such as the poor conditions in which many animals are housed, and it is easy to see why people choose not to eat animals or animal by-products. Horrible practices like debeaking, dehorning, castration, and tail docking are routinely carried out in the meat industry. Animals are confined in crowded conditions and are often given hormones to increase production and growth rate. And fishing leads to the death of sea animals that are unintentionally caught and then discarded.

For the Earth

In 2006, the Food and Agriculture Organization of the United Nations released an important report, "Livestock's Long Shadow: Environmental Issues and Options," assessing livestock's effect on the environment. Livestock production was shown to have a serious effect on land degradation, climate change, air pollution, water shortage and pollution, and the loss of biodiversity. The report concluded that the livestock sector is responsible for a greater production of greenhouse gas than automobiles and other forms of transportation. Livestock also produce almost two-thirds of ammonia emissions, a significant contributor to acid rain.

According to the report, in the United States "livestock are responsible for an estimated 55 percent of erosion and sediment, 37 percent of pesticide use, [and] 50 percent of antibiotic use."

For Personal Health

Besides planetary health and health for animals, many vegans recognize significant health benefits from their dietary choices. Vegan diets do not contain cholesterol and are typically low in saturated fats, making them heart-healthy diets. Vegans frequently eat generous amounts of fiber-containing foods like beans, whole grains, and fruits and vegetables. As a group, vegans and vegetarians tend to be leaner than nonvegans and nonvegetarians. Vegan diets have been used to treat medical conditions, including heart disease and type 2 diabetes.

Other Reasons

While ethics, the environment, and health are the most commonly cited reasons for choosing to be vegan, other motives are also identified. Some people choose to be vegan for reasons related to world hunger. Some become vegan because their loved ones are vegan. Some find a vegan diet to be very economical and choose it as a money-saving technique. Some people want to avoid the hormones and other additives that are frequently introduced into animal products. Some look at veganism as a part of an overall lifestyle committed to nonviolence.

Whatever your reason is for becoming vegan, it's important not to judge other people. How people choose to follow a vegan diet can vary according to their personal beliefs, background, reasons for being vegan, and knowledge level. Be aware that no one is perfect, try to do your best, and avoid being judgmental of others. That's how you can use your lifestyle to promote a more humane and caring world.

Health Benefits of Being Vegan

According to the previously mentioned 2016 position paper on vegetarian diets by the Academy of Nutrition and Dietetics, "appropriately planned vegetarian, including vegan, diets are healthful, nutritionally adequate, and may provide health benefits in the prevention and treatment of certain diseases." There are significant health advantages associated with both vegan and other types of vegetarian diets.

For example, a 2007 study published by the Brazilian Society of Cardiology found that vegetarians and vegans had lower levels of triglycerides and total and LDL cholesterol in their blood compared to omnivores. LDL cholesterol is often referred to as "bad" cholesterol because it is associated with a higher risk of heart disease. When compared to vegetarians who ate eggs and dairy products, vegans had the lowest levels of triglycerides and total and LDL cholesterol.

According to a 2009 *Diabetes Care* article, one significant health advantage for vegans is that they tend to have lower body weights than either other vegetarians or meat eaters. Since being overweight increases the risk of developing many chronic diseases, including heart disease, type 2 diabetes, high blood pressure, and even breast cancer, the lower average weight seen in vegans is a definite plus.

High blood pressure also increases the risk of developing heart disease and of having a stroke. Vegans tend to have lower blood pressure than meat eaters and a lower risk of developing hypertension (high blood pressure).

Several studies have used vegan or near-vegan diets to treat people with heart disease. Results have been very positive in terms of modifying risk factors like obesity and LDL cholesterol levels.

Vegetarians tend to have a lower overall risk of developing cancers than meat eaters. Research on vegans is limited. A 2015 study by Loma Linda University found that vegans had a lower risk of prostate cancer than did other vegetarians, and a 2013 study also from Loma Linda University found that vegans had a lower risk of breast, uterine, and ovarian cancer. Overall, vegans experienced modest risk reduction (14 percent) for all cancer, but not significant for vegetarians. Being a vegetarian reduced the risk of cancer of the gastrointestinal tract by 24 percent.

As noted in a 2013 study by Loma Linda University researchers, vegans also have lower rates of type 2 diabetes. Type 2 diabetes is the most common form of diabetes. Risk factors for type 2 diabetes include a poor diet, excess weight, and little exercise. Low-fat vegan diets have been successfully used to treat type 2 diabetes. Vegetarians are half as likely to develop metabolic syndrome as nonvegetarians.

Chapter 2

Getting Ready for Your Vegan Pregnancy

Pregnancy is a time of big changes for you and your family. It's so exciting to think about having a new family member! There's a lot to learn as you prepare for parenthood, so be patient with yourself. Even before you're pregnant, you can take some positive steps to ensure that you're as healthy as possible. Eating well, exercising regularly, and evaluating your lifestyle practices and physical and emotional health are ways to get ready. You can also identify a healthcare provider you trust who will support you.

Optimizing Your Weight

If you are planning to have a baby, the American College of Obstetricians and Gynecologists (ACOG) recommends you try to reach a healthy weight before becoming pregnant. If you are slightly underweight, gaining a few pounds can help increase the odds that you will become pregnant as well as reduce the risk of having a baby who is too small and has problems after birth. If you are overweight, losing weight before becoming pregnant can help reduce your risk of gestational diabetes, high blood pressure, preeclampsia, and cesarean section. Babies whose moms are overweight are at higher risk for developing macrosomia, a body weight of 8 pounds, 13 ounces (4,000 grams) or more, which could make it difficult to pass through the birth canal. Macrosomia also increases the risk of childhood obesity. Since weight loss is not usually recommended during pregnancy, it makes sense to drop a few pounds before becoming pregnant.

If You Need to Gain Weight

As a group, vegetarians and vegans both weigh less than nonvegetarians and nonvegans. That's not to say that vegans don't come in every body shape and size possible, but simply that it's more likely you'll weigh somewhat less if you're following a vegan diet. Refer to the following table to see if your prepregnancy weight is considered underweight. If it is, try to gain a few pounds before you become pregnant.

The following are a few ideas you can use to add more calories to your diet, and more calories = weight gain.

- **Be sure you're eating often.** Often means breakfast, lunch, dinner, and one or more substantial snacks. A snack can be as simple as a piece of fruit and a handful of nuts, and breakfast can be a bowl of whole-grain cereal with fruit and soy milk.
- **Make beverages count.** Drink smoothies, shakes, fruit or vegetable juices, and hot chocolate (made with fortified soy milk). Water, coffee, and tea are wonderful calorie-free beverages, but when you're trying to gain weight, drink some other beverages also. You will want to limit your caffeine intake.
- **Indulge a bit.** Sure, you want to eat a healthy diet, but when you're trying to gain a bit of weight, treat yourself to some higher-calorie foods—a scoop of

nondairy frozen dessert, a vegan cookie or muffin, a granola bar, a handful of trail mix, for instance.

- **Save the salad for last.** Have you ever noticed that when you eat a large salad, suddenly you're not that hungry anymore? It's a great strategy for weight loss, but if you're trying to gain weight, don't fill up on bulky low-calorie foods before you've had a chance to eat other higher-calorie foods.
- **Add some oils, nuts, and other high-fat foods.** Ounce for ounce, foods made up mostly of fat are higher-calorie foods than starches or protein. Take advantage of this fact and sauté vegetables in olive oil, spread vegan margarine or peanut butter on your breakfast bagel, and add a creamy vegan dressing to your salad.

If your height is	If your prepregnancy weight is less than this, you are considered underweight
4'10"	91 pounds
4'11"	94 pounds
5'0"	97 pounds
5'1"	100 pounds
5'2"	104 pounds
5'3"	107 pounds
5'4"	110 pounds
5'5"	114 pounds
5'6"	118 pounds
5'7"	121 pounds
5'8"	125 pounds
5'9"	128 pounds
5'10"	132 pounds
5'11"	136 pounds
6'0"	140 pounds

And, if you're trying to gain a bit of weight before becoming pregnant, take a look at your exercise habits. Exercise is great (more about this soon), but it's probably not the time to spend several hours each day exercising since you'll need to eat even more to compensate for the calories you expend when you exercise.

If You Need to Lose Weight

Although many vegans are of average weight, there are definitely vegans whose weight is higher than that recommended. If you're in that category, spending a few months focusing on diet and exercise can provide significant benefits in terms of your upcoming pregnancy. Of course, if you're already pregnant, it's not the time to go on a weight-reduction diet.

If your height is	If your prepregnancy weight is more than this, you are considered overweight
4'10"	119 pounds
4'11"	124 pounds
5'0"	128 pounds
5'1"	132 pounds
5'2"	136 pounds
5'3"	141 pounds
5'4"	145 pounds
5'5"	150 pounds
5'6"	155 pounds
5'7"	159 pounds
5'8"	164 pounds
5'9"	169 pounds
5'10"	174 pounds
5'11"	179 pounds
6'0"	184 pounds

To reach a healthy weight before pregnancy, focus on healthy foods. Eat plenty of fruits, vegetables, and whole grains every day along with moderate amounts of dried beans and soy products. Limit high-calorie, low-nutrient foods like sweets, sodas, oils, margarine, snack foods, and salad dressings. Remember, improvements that you make with your eating habits now will make it even easier to have a good diet during pregnancy.

You may find it helpful to discuss a weight-reduction diet with a registered dietitian (RD), a food and nutrition expert who has met specific academic and professional requirements to qualify for the RD credential.

In addition to the RD credential, your nutrition advisor may have other credentials. Many states have regulatory laws for dietitians and nutrition practitioners, so you may see credentials like LD (licensed dietitian) or LN (licensed nutritionist). You can find an RD by contacting the Academy of Nutrition and Dietetics (see Appendix A for contact information). Your healthcare provider or local hospital may also be able to recommend an RD in your area.

According to the Academy of Nutrition and Dietetics, requirements for being an RD include a minimum of a bachelor's degree from an approved college or university and an accredited preprofessional experience program. RDs must successfully complete a rigorous professional-level exam and must maintain ongoing continuing education to maintain their credential. Some RDs hold advanced degrees and additional certifications in specialized areas of practice.

Folic Acid and Vitamin B$_{12}$

Folic acid (folate) and vitamin B$_{12}$ are two important vitamins to be aware of even before you become pregnant. Folic acid is an issue for all women contemplating pregnancy. Since vegans must get vitamin B$_{12}$ from fortified foods or supplements, it's important to make sure that you are choosing foods or a vitamin pill that provide this essential nutrient.

Folic acid significantly lowers your baby's risk of developing neural tube defects (birth defects of the brain and spinal cord, such as spina bifida and anencephaly). Because the neural tube forms during the first four weeks of pregnancy, before many women even realize they are pregnant, the Centers for Disease Control and Prevention (CDC) recommends that all women of childbearing age do one of the following:

- Take a vitamin that has folic acid in it every day. This can be either a folic acid supplement or a multivitamin. Most multivitamins sold in the United States have 400–800 micrograms of folic acid, the amount nonpregnant women need each day. Check the label of the vitamin to make sure that it contains at least 100 percent of the daily value of folic acid. For reference, Percent Daily Value (DV) is a guide to the nutrients in one serving of food. DVs are based on a 2,000-calorie diet for healthy adults. Another thing to be aware of is the MTHFR gene. This is a gene coding for folic acid metabolism. If women have certain mutations of this gene, it may predispose them to miscarriage and other problems. It is easy to check for with a simple blood test or cheek swab. While it may be slightly controversial at the moment, in the future it may become more and more prevalent. For more information visit Genetics Home Reference (https://ghr.nlm.nih.gov).
- Eat a bowl of breakfast cereal or other fortified food that has at least 100 percent of the DV of folic acid every day. Check the label on the side of the cereal box to make sure that it has at least 100 percent next to folic acid. Use of a vitamin or a fortified food containing at least 100 percent of the DV for folic acid, or a combination of both, should be a daily practice throughout pregnancy. In addition, you can get some folic acid from other foods that you eat. Folic acid is added to breads, cereal, pasta, rice, and flour and is found naturally in leafy dark-green vegetables, citrus fruits and juices, and beans. Because the amounts in foods vary and it may be hard to get all of the folic acid you need from food sources alone, you should use either a supplement or a fortified breakfast cereal daily.

Each year, approximately three thousand babies are born with neural tube defects. According to the CDC resource guide, up to 70 percent of these defects could be prevented by adequate intake of folic acid, yet according to a 2017 March of Dimes survey, less than 50 percent of American women of childbearing age (ages eighteen to forty-five) take a daily multivitamin containing folic acid to ensure they meet the daily requirements.

Vitamin B_{12} plays an important role in the development of the baby's brain and nervous system. Vegans must get vitamin B_{12} from foods fortified with this nutrient or from supplements containing vitamin B_{12}. Foods that may be fortified with vitamin B_{12} include:

- Soy milk, rice milk, and other commercial plant milks
- Meat analogues (veggie "meats")
- Breakfast cereals
- Nutritional yeast

Since vitamin B_{12} plays such an important role in the baby's development (as well as being important for your health), making sure you are accustomed to using a daily, reliable source of vitamin B_{12} before becoming pregnant is a smart, caring idea. Before you are pregnant, you need 2.4 micrograms of vitamin B_{12} daily; once you're pregnant, the amount increases to 2.6 micrograms. Check the label to make sure the fortified food or supplement supplies at least this amount of vitamin B_{12}.

Remember, you need only small amounts of both folic acid and vitamin B_{12}, but they are both essential vitamins. One easy way to make sure you're getting enough is to take a daily multivitamin that provides 400–800 micrograms of folic acid and at least 2.4 micrograms (2.6 micrograms after you are pregnant) of vitamin B_{12}.

Some websites claim there are nonanimal sources of vitamin B_{12} besides fortified foods or supplements. Miso, sauerkraut, shiitake mushrooms, tempeh, sourdough bread, sea vegetables, spirulina (algae), soybeans, and umeboshi plums have all been proposed as good sources of vitamin B_{12}. When tested, however, these foods are not actually reliable sources and may contain a vitamin B_{12} analogue (something that looks like vitamin B_{12} but isn't) that can interfere with the vitamin's absorption from other foods. Your baby's health is too important—choose reliable fortified foods or supplements as your vitamin B_{12} sources.

Finding a Healthcare Provider

Even if you have a model pregnancy, you will be seeing a lot of your healthcare provider over the next nine months. ACOG recommends that women see their provider every four weeks through the first twenty-eight weeks of pregnancy (about the first seven months). After week twenty-eight, the visits will increase to once every two to three weeks until week thirty-six, after which you'll be paying your doctor or midwife a weekly visit until your baby arrives. If you have any conditions that put you in a high-risk category (such as diabetes or history of preterm labor), your provider may want to see you more frequently to monitor your progress.

The Options

So who should guide you on this odyssey of birth? If you currently see a gynecologist or family practice doctor who also has an obstetric practice, she may be a good choice. If you don't have that choice or would like to explore your options, consider:

- An ob-gyn: An obstetrician and gynecologist is a medical doctor (MD) who has received specialized training in women's health and reproductive medicine.
- A perinatologist: If you have a chronic health condition, you may see a perinatologist—an ob-gyn who specializes in overseeing high-risk pregnancies.
- A midwife: Certified nurse-midwives are licensed to practice in all fifty states. They provide patient-focused care throughout pregnancy, labor, and delivery.
- A nurse practitioner: A nurse practitioner (NP) is a registered nurse (RN) with advanced medical education and training (at minimum, a master's degree).
- A combination of practitioners: Some obstetric practices blend midwives, NPs, and MDs, with the choice (or sometimes the requirement) of seeing one or more of these throughout your pregnancy.

Networking and Referrals

Finding Dr. Right may seem like a monumental task. After all, this is the person you're entrusting your pregnancy and childbirth to. Unless you're paying completely out of pocket for all prenatal care, labor, and delivery expenses, your first consideration is probably your health insurance coverage. If you are part of a managed-care organization, your insurer may require that you see someone within its provider network. Getting a current copy of the network directory, if one is available, can help you narrow down your choices by coverage and location.

ACOG can help you find a physician (all ACOG fellows are board-certified ob-gyns) in your area. To find a nurse-midwife, contact the American College of Nurse-Midwives. (See Appendix A for contact information for both of these organizations.)

Many women choose a physician solely for logistical reasons (for example, insurance will cover all of his fees or she's near your place of work). Although money and convenience are important factors, these won't mean much if you aren't happy with the care you receive and the role the physician ultimately plays in your pregnancy and birth. Whether your first or your fifth, this pregnancy is a onetime event, and you deserve the best support in seeing it through. Talk to the experts—girlfriends and other women you know and trust—and get referrals. Be aware, of course, that not everyone looks for the same thing in a healthcare provider; what one woman emphasizes, you may downplay.

If you've just moved to a new area or simply don't know any moms or moms-to-be, there are other referral options available. The licensing authority in your area (the state or county medical board) can typically provide you with references for local practitioners. You may also try the patient services department or labor and delivery programs of nearby hospitals and/or birthing centers. Most medical centers will be happy to offer you several provider referrals, and you can get information on their facilities in the process. If you're especially interested in finding a vegan-friendly healthcare provider, contact local vegetarian or vegan groups to find out if others are aware of such local practitioners.

Ask the Right Questions

Once you've collected names and phone numbers, narrowed down your list of potential providers, and verified that they accept (and are accepted by) your health insurance plan, it's time to do some legwork. Sit down with your partner and talk about your biggest questions, concerns, and expectations. Then compile a list of provider interview questions. Some issues to consider:

- **What are the costs and payment options?** If your health plan doesn't provide full coverage, find out how much the remaining fees will run and whether installment plans are available.
- **Who will deliver my baby?** Will the doctor or midwife you select deliver your child or another provider in the practice, depending on when the baby arrives? If your provider works alone, find out who covers his patients during vacations and emergencies.
- **Whom will I see during office visits?** Since group practices typically share delivery responsibilities, you might want to ask about rotating your prenatal appointments among all the providers in the group so you'll see a familiar face in the delivery room when the big day arrives.
- **What is your philosophy on routine IVs, episiotomies, labor induction, pain relief, and other interventions in the birth process?** If you have certain expectations regarding medical interventions during labor and delivery, you should lay them out now.
- **What hospital or birthing center will I go to?** Find out where the provider has hospital privileges and obtain more information on that facility's programs and policies, if possible. Is a neonatal unit available if problems arise after the baby's birth? Many hospitals offer tours of their labor and delivery rooms for expectant parents.
- **What is your policy on birth plans?** Will the provider work with you to create and, more importantly, follow a birth plan? Will the plan be signed and become part of your permanent chart in case she is off duty during the birth?
- **How are phone calls handled if I have a health concern or question?** Most obstetric practices have some sort of triage (or prioritizing) system in place for patient phone calls. Ask how quickly calls are returned and what system the practice has in place for handling night and weekend patient calls.

Some providers have the staff to answer these sorts of inquiries over the phone, while others might schedule a face-to-face appointment with your prospective doctor or midwife. Either way, make sure that all your questions are answered to your satisfaction so you can make a fully informed choice.

Comfort and Communication

As with any good relationship, communication is essential between patients and their providers. Does the provider encourage your questions, answer them thoroughly, and really listen to your concerns? Does he make sure all your questions are answered before concluding the appointment? Are the nursing and administrative staff attentive to patients' needs and willing to answer questions as well?

Good healthcare is a partnership or, more accurately, a team effort. Although ultimately you call the shots (it's your body and your baby, after all), your provider serves as your coach and trainer, giving you the support and training you need to reach the finish line. If your doctor doesn't listen to your needs in the first place, she won't be able to meet them. Remember as well that communication works both ways. Your provider has likely been around the block a few times and has a wealth of useful information to offer you, particularly if you're a rookie at this baby game.

Gender may also be an issue for you. Some women feel more at ease with a female physician because of communication style and the fact that the physician may have been through pregnancy herself. Other women prefer a male doctor for various reasons. Making an issue of gender may seem silly or, at worst, discriminatory and hypocritical. The subject is serious enough to merit a number of clinical studies and patient surveys in the medical literature both for and against a clear gender preference. The bottom line is that you are the one who has to live with your provider choice for the next nine months, and to spend it feeling awkward, stressed, and inhibited—emotions that can ultimately have a negative effect on your pregnancy—is not healthy. Whatever your choice, make sure it's one you'll be comfortable with.

Lastly, have the tough talk with your provider sooner rather than later. It's important to discuss the risks of birth early on in your pregnancy with your provider. For example, per the CDC, nearly 1.3 million babies (about one out of every three) born in the US in 2016 were delivered via cesarean section. Have a frank discussion with your provider about how common situations like these will be handled to make sure you are all on the same page.

Talking to Your Healthcare Provider about Your Vegan Diet

You may be fortunate enough to find a healthcare provider who is either vegan or very knowledgeable about vegan diets. If so, that's wonderful. It's more likely, though, given the number of vegans in the United States, that your practitioner has only general knowledge of vegan diets. This is a great opportunity to educate your provider so that you can work together to ensure a healthy pregnancy.

You may wonder if you should even mention your vegan diet at all. In the spirit of open communication and honesty, you should. Saying something like "I've been vegan for the past five years and feel pretty comfortable with my diet" lets your doctor know that you've been doing this for a while and that you're confident about your choice. If you've worked with an RD (or plan to do so), mention this.

Your healthcare provider may smile, say something positive ("Great! Thanks for letting me know. Some of my healthiest patients are vegans."), and move on. He may ask you for more details like which foods you avoid or where you get various nutrients. Come prepared (but not defensive). Describe your diet in simple, positive terms: "I eat beans, whole grains, nuts, fruits, and vegetables. I don't eat meat, fish, poultry, eggs, or dairy products." Think about where you get some key nutrients like protein, vitamin B_{12}, calcium, iron, and vitamin D (see upcoming chapters for details) and be ready to answer questions. This could be an opportunity to fine-tune your dietary choices as you prepare for pregnancy.

If you'd like to go a bit further, give your healthcare provider a brief update on vegan diets: "I recently read that the Academy of Nutrition and Dietetics said well-planned vegan diets were fine for pregnant women." Offer to share references. Provide your doctor with a link to the academy's position paper on vegetarian diets or other resources. Bring in this book and share it with your doctor. By keeping the tone positive, upbeat, and informational, you're letting your provider know that you're willing to work as a partner and that you're knowledgeable about your diet.

If, despite your best efforts, your potential provider continues to disparage vegan diets, it may be time to courteously end the visit and consider whether or not this is the right provider for you.

Exercising Your Body

Women often wonder whether or not they should start, stop, increase, or decrease their exercise routines if they're trying to get pregnant. In most cases, regular exercise before getting pregnant is encouraged. Plenty of exercise promotes good health throughout your life. Exercise can help you lose a few pounds if you need to before becoming pregnant. Your ability to stay active throughout your pregnancy depends on your health and activity level before pregnancy.

If you're just starting out with exercising, start with something simple like walking, swimming, or biking. If you are not used to a lot of exercise, check with your doctor about safety guidelines and don't overdo it at first. Gradually increase both the time and intensity of your exercise.

Part 2

What to Eat for a Healthy Pregnancy

Chapter 3

The Need for Protein

What nutrition question are vegans asked most often? If you guessed, "Where do you get protein?" or something similar, you're probably right. People mistakenly believe that you can only get enough protein from a diet heavy on beef, pork, chicken, fish, dairy products, and eggs with added protein powder "just to be sure." Not to worry. Most people, vegans included, get plenty of protein, even when their protein needs are higher because of strenuous exercise or, more relevantly, being pregnant.

How Much Protein Do You Need?

The word *protein* comes from the Greek word *proteios*, meaning "primary." Perhaps this word was chosen because of protein's primary role in the body. Proteins are responsible for everything from the structure of your muscles and bones to the proper function of your immune system to food digestion. Additionally, many hormones are made from protein, and adequate protein helps promote healthy skin, hair, and nails. In pregnancy, extra protein is needed to support your baby's growth—building bones and muscles, for example. You also need extra protein as your blood volume increases and your breasts and uterus enlarge.

> During pregnancy, you'll gain a bit more than 2 pounds of protein. About a pound of this is accounted for by your baby's muscle, hair, skin, bones, teeth, and internal organs. The other pound or so is added to your usual body protein content.

Before you were pregnant, you needed around 0.4 grams of protein for every pound that you weighed. To do the math, take your prepregnancy weight in pounds and multiply by 0.4—that's how much protein you needed before you were pregnant. For instance, if you weighed 120 pounds, you'd multiply 120 by 0.4 (calculators allowed, this is not a test!) and get 48 grams of protein.

Protein Needs in Pregnancy

Even early in your pregnancy, protein needs increase to support changes to your body and your baby's growth. You need about 25 grams of protein a day more than you did before you were pregnant. Simply take the amount of protein recommended before pregnancy (0.4 times your prepregnancy weight) and add 25 grams. So for instance, if you weighed 120 pounds before pregnancy, you'd multiply 120 by 0.4 and then add 25 for a total of 73 grams of protein. That's how much daily protein (in grams) is recommended. This amount is about 50 percent higher than protein recommendations for nonpregnant women.

If you're lucky enough to be expecting twins, you'll need even extra protein. After all, instead of one baby, you have two on the way. Moms of twins should add

50 grams of protein to their prepregnancy protein needs. So, if you calculated your protein needs before you were pregnant as 48 grams a day, you'd add 50 grams for a total of 98 grams of protein to aim for.

Some vegan nutrition experts recommend that vegans get slightly more protein than nonvegans. Their rationale is that vegan protein sources like beans and whole grains are harder to digest. They suggest about 10 percent more protein for vegans. This amount is pretty small and is nothing to be concerned about. If you want to calculate, multiply your protein recommendation by 1.1.

Vegan Protein Sources

The list of vegan foods that don't contain protein is a much shorter list than those foods that do supply protein. Foods that provide protein include all varieties of beans from adzuki to yellow, grains, nuts and seeds, nut butters and seed butters, vegetables, potatoes, soy foods, meat analogues (products made to resemble meats), and seitan (wheat "meat"). The short list of poor sources of protein is just that: short.

Foods and ingredients that are not good sources of protein include:

- Fats and oils—margarine, olive oil, canola oil, other oils, most salad dressings
- Sugar and other sweeteners—maple syrup, molasses, agave nectar
- Soft drinks, coffee, tea
- Herbs and spices—the amounts you eat are too small to provide much protein
- Fruits—note that fruits are great foods; they're just not good protein sources
- Alcohol—but you're not drinking that anyway, right?

So unless you're feasting on hard candy, fried bananas, wine coolers, and the like for every meal, every day, chances are that you're getting a good amount of protein.

Another issue to be aware of is whether you are getting enough calories. Ideally, you're gaining weight at the rate that you should for pregnancy. If you are, chances are that you're getting enough calories. Not gaining weight could mean you're eating fewer calories than you need, which means that protein is being used mainly to keep your body functions going instead of being used to build your baby's muscles.

When you go for a routine prenatal visit to your doctor, your urine will be tested for protein. This is mainly a test for preeclampsia, urinary tract infection, and kidney function. This test does not provide information about how much protein is in your diet.

Your protein intake will naturally increase as you eat more food when you are pregnant, especially if you focus on foods that are good sources of protein.

How Much Protein Are You Eating?

You probably aren't going to approach each meal with a calculator in hand to make sure that you're meeting your protein needs. Chances are you don't even need to be concerned about protein. An occasional spot check, however, can provide some peace of mind. Here's how to do it. First, write down everything you ate on a typical day and how much you ate of each food. Then, use an online nutrition program to calculate how much protein you ate. One recommended website is www.webmd.com/diet/healthtool-food-calorie-counter.

Use food labels to see how much protein is in foods that aren't in an online database. Refer to recommendations in this chapter for protein intake in pregnancy, and compare your protein needs to the amount of protein in your diet and make any adjustments needed.

Remember, this is just one day. If you eat much the same from one day to the next, you can be pretty confident that your results provide a reliable picture of your diet. If your eating habits vary widely, make sure that your diet has several good sources of protein every day.

Protein in Vegan Foods

Some vegan foods that are especially high in protein are soybeans, lentils, and tempeh. These foods have 18 or more grams of protein in a serving—a cup of soybeans or lentils or 4 ounces of tempeh. Other foods that provide generous amounts of protein (10–20 grams per serving) include tofu, veggie burgers, and cooked dried beans. Soy milk, peanut butter, soy yogurt, and quinoa are all good sources of protein as well. Vegetables, whole grains, pasta, almond butter, and nuts and seeds are other good foods to add to your protein intake.

There are some easy ways to incorporate good sources of protein into your daily meal plan. These are all highly nutritious foods, so by adding them you're adding not just protein but a host of vitamins and minerals as well.

AT BREAKFAST

- Spread some peanut butter or other nut butter on your toast or bagel; peanut butter can even top oatmeal—add a spoonful of jelly for PB and J oatmeal.
- Blend soft or silken tofu with soy milk and fruit (fresh, frozen, or canned) for a quick smoothie.
- Use soy milk in place of water to prepare hot cereals.
- Mix things up with a bowl of quinoa instead of oatmeal.
- Replace water or other liquids in your favorite muffin and pancake recipes with soy milk.
- On more leisurely mornings, try a tofu scramble or quiche for breakfast.

AT LUNCH

- Toss some chickpeas or black beans with your salad.
- Use a flavored hummus in place of mayo as a savory sandwich spread.
- Prepare a vegan cream soup with soy milk.
- Add extra crunch to a peanut butter sandwich by sprinkling on coarsely chopped peanuts or other nuts.
- Pack protein-rich leftovers to reheat at lunchtime.

AT DINNER

- Purée white beans or soft tofu with your favorite tomato sauce and serve over whole-grain pasta.

- Top baked potatoes with a spoonful of plain soy yogurt and some chopped chives.
- Top rice, pasta, or vegetables with a peanut sauce (homemade or purchased).
- Add chickpeas or vegan pepperoni to takeout or homemade veggie no-cheese pizza.
- Experiment with quinoa in dishes that use rice or other grains.
- Toss vegan stir-fry strips or homemade seitan with stir-fried vegetables.

FOR SNACKS

- Make a batch of trail mix using a variety of nuts and dried fruits. Add soy nuts for a protein boost.
- Spread apple or pear slices with nut butters.
- Dip baby carrots and jicama strips into hummus or refried beans.
- Try different brands of vegan energy bars until you find one or more that suit you.
- Eat breakfast for a snack by having a bowl of cold cereal with soy milk.

If you like to bake, you can boost the protein in breads and muffins by adding soy flour. For yeast-raised breads, put 2 tablespoons of soy flour in your 1-cup measuring cup and then fill the cup with the flour your recipe calls for. Repeat until you've measured all of the recipe's flour. Since soy flour does not contain gluten, which gives bread its structure, it cannot completely replace wheat flour. For quick breads or muffins, replace up to a quarter of the flour with soy flour.

You'll probably think of even more ways to add protein-rich soy products, beans, seitan, nuts, and nut butters to your meals and snacks.

Protein Combining

Have you ever been asked if you "combine" proteins? Protein combining is based on the fact that humans need certain amino acids in order to build each type of protein. For example, the protein found in your hair would use a different mixture of amino acids than the protein found in your muscles. Fortunately, your body is able to store amino acids from one meal to the next, so it's not necessary to eat perfect amounts of amino acids at every meal.

There are nine amino acids your body cannot make, so you have to get them from foods. Some vegan foods contain generous amounts of all nine essential amino acids. These foods include soy products (soybeans, tofu, tempeh, and soy milk); quinoa; and hemp seed. Other foods still provide some of each essential amino acid; they may be higher in one and lower in another compared to the so-called reference proteins (like cow's milk and eggs).

By eating a variety of foods over the entire day, you can eliminate the need to worry about strict protein combining. The higher levels of the amino acid lysine in the bean dip you eat for a snack will supplement breakfast's whole-wheat toast that doesn't have that much lysine. In turn, whole-wheat toast can provide a boost in methionine, an amino acid that is lower in beans. Experienced vegans don't even think about protein combining. They simply eat a variety of good sources of protein like beans, grains, nuts, and soy products over the course of the day.

Food Cravings

Some vegan moms-to-be report protein cravings. All of a sudden, a committed vegan is craving steak or broiled salmon. If this happens to you, you may wonder if it indicates a dietary deficiency. Chances are good that it doesn't. Scientists don't really understand why some people experience cravings for certain foods, but reports, like one found in *Scientific American*, state that the food being craved has no relationship to nutritional status.

So how do you explain the craving for a juicy burger or a wedge of cheese? It may simply be that you've been conditioned to equate protein, especially meat or dairy products, with health. In pregnancy, when you're trying to do everything right for your baby, those old habits kick in and you may question whether or not you're getting what you need. Step back and look at what you are eating. It may even be worthwhile in terms of peace of mind to make an appointment with an RD who is knowledgeable about vegan nutrition. He can look at your eating habits and let you know if you need to make any adjustments to get enough protein on your vegan diet. Chances are that you won't need to make changes, but it is reassuring to have another set of eyes look at what you're eating.

Cravings may also be for comfort, rather than food. When you're dreaming of your mom's meatloaf, maybe you're really longing for the good old days when your biggest responsibility was walking the dog or setting the table. If that's the case, try some alternative comfort measures instead of Mom's meatloaf recipe. Order a vegan take-out meal, soak in a hot tub, or call a friend.

Some women find that eating a vegan meat look-alike helps them cope with their cravings. Others report success with eating something salty or a bit fatty, like a handful of salted nuts or a spoonful of hummus, for instance.

Food cravings, and not just for higher-protein foods, are common in pregnancy. Whether it's the stereotypical pickles and ice cream or something else, you may find yourself really wanting a certain food, not necessarily something you would usually eat. Some researchers believe that these kinds of cravings are due to hormonal changes that accompany pregnancy. These hormone shifts lead to an intensified sense of smell. Since smell is related to taste, there may be some connection among smells, tastes, and cravings. You may find that your cravings change from day to day and even from one pregnancy to the next.

You may also find yourself craving fresh fruit or vegetables. If that's the case, keep the refrigerator stocked with these healthy snacks. If, however, you find that your cravings are leading to frequent junk-food binges, it's time for some coping tips.

- Low blood sugar may trigger cravings. Try to avoid precipitous drops in your blood sugar levels by eating frequent small meals and snacks.
- Emotional stress may also play a role. Ask yourself if this is really a craving or a reaction to stress or boredom. Think of coping mechanisms like taking a walk or doing some gentle yoga.
- Sometimes a craving can be satisfied by eating a bite or two of the food you're fixated on. Eat a bite and then do something else. And don't leave the open bag of chips on the counter!
- Try to think of a healthier substitute for the food you crave. If you're craving French fries, make oven-baked fries; instead of a bag of chocolate chips, try a cup of hot cocoa.

Cravings will pass with time. It's unlikely that after your baby is born you'll still be longing for peanut butter and barbecue potato chip sandwiches!

Protein Myths

There are tons of myths about protein out there. From rumors that unless you eat meat you're in danger of protein deficiency to the mistaken notion that proteins have to be carefully combined, there is a lot of misinformation about protein. Hopefully, you're already convinced that protein adequacy is entirely possible on a vegan diet and that careful meal-based protein combining is not necessary. There are other myths about protein that you may encounter.

Plant Proteins Are Incomplete

The myth that plant proteins are incomplete, or somehow inferior to animal proteins, refers to the amino acids in plant proteins. While protein from plants contains all of the nine essential amino acids, some amino acids may be present in lower amounts in plant proteins than in animal-derived protein. Eating a variety of plant protein sources makes it likely, however, that you'll get the amount of amino acids that you need.

Vegans Need to Use Protein Supplements

Protein supplements come in different forms, most commonly powders that are mixed with water or other liquids. Vegan protein supplements do exist and are usually based on soy, rice, or hemp protein. If you are eating a varied vegan diet that includes good sources of protein, it's unlikely that any protein supplement is needed. Of course, if you have a number of food restrictions because of allergies or intolerances or have especially high protein needs because of a medical condition, your RD may suggest using protein supplements. For most vegan women, however, they are an unnecessary expense.

Exercising Increases Your Protein Needs

The area of protein needs with strenuous exercise is a controversial one. Some research suggests that people engaging in strenuous exercise have somewhat higher protein needs while other research does not support any increase in protein. The kind of strenuous exercise that might affect protein needs is not the kind that you are doing while pregnant. Protein needs are higher for those who are training for a fast-paced marathon or doing intensive weight lifting for bodybuilding purposes. Your protein needs are already somewhat higher in the second and third trimesters of your pregnancy; the exercise you participate in during pregnancy—walking, biking, swimming, or even running—should not be strenuous enough to markedly increase your protein needs above those of pregnancy.

Vegan Etiquette: When Others Ask about Protein

You're at a restaurant with your coworkers and someone remembers that you're vegan. They also know you're pregnant. With a concerned look, they ask, "Now that you're pregnant, how are you going to be able to get enough protein on a vegan diet?" Remember, it's likely that:

- They are genuinely concerned
- They know next to nothing about vegan nutrition
- Their eyes will start to glaze over if your answer takes more than a minute or two
- They really want reassurance that you're on top of things and aren't doing anything harmful

Keep your answer brief, calm, friendly, and positive. Even if you've answered this question hundreds of times, simply say something like, "I've been reading some excellent books about vegan nutrition just to make sure I'm doing everything right. I get the protein I need from beans, grains, soy products, nuts, and vegetables." And then change the subject: "I'm having the veggie burger with a baked potato. How about you?"

Chapter 4

The Importance of Iron and Zinc

The requirements for iron and zinc are very small (think milligrams), but these minerals play important roles in your baby's development. Vegans face the challenge of compensating for reduced absorption of iron and zinc from plant foods. On the positive side, plants also contain absorption-boosting substances. Many women will be advised by their healthcare provider to take iron pills during pregnancy because it is so challenging for most women (not just vegans) to get enough iron solely from food at this time of high iron needs.

Iron Needs

Iron's major role is to help red blood cells deliver oxygen throughout your body. When you are pregnant, iron also helps deliver oxygen to your baby. A woman's need for iron increases dramatically in pregnancy, especially in the second and third trimesters. In pregnancy, your body's blood supply actually increases 40–50 percent. In order to make this extra blood, you need more iron than you do when you're not pregnant. Your unborn baby is also storing iron that will last for the first few months of life outside your womb. Baby takes what she needs from your store of iron first, so she won't suffer unless you are very low in iron. However, you can end up with iron-deficiency anemia.

After your baby is born, your iron needs go down dramatically. Not only are you not making extra blood or supporting your baby's growth anymore, but you also won't be having menstrual periods for a little while, which means you're not losing iron each month in menstrual flow.

Pregnancy does boost the amount of iron that you absorb, especially in the second trimester. Eating foods that contain plenty of iron lets you take advantage of this natural increase in iron absorption. Nonvegetarians and nonvegans don't benefit as much from the increased iron absorption later in pregnancy, since only the nonheme form of iron is better absorbed.

Iron for Vegans

Recommendations for iron are higher for vegetarians than for nonvegetarians. This is because all of the iron in vegetarian diets is found in a form called *nonheme* iron, which is not as well absorbed as some of the iron found in meat. Part of the iron in meat is in a form called *heme* iron, which is especially well absorbed.

According to sources, including the National Institutes of Health, vegetarians need 1.8 times more iron than nonvegetarians. Vegan diets can be particularly high in substances that interfere with iron absorption. That's not to say, of course, that you can't get the iron you need on a vegan and vegetarian diet. It's possible, with smart food choices, for vegan women to meet the vegetarian Recommended Dietary Allowance (RDA) for nonpregnant women of 32 milligrams of iron per day. When you add in the higher iron needs that go with pregnancy, however, many women find that taking a daily iron pill, along with choosing high-iron foods, is exactly what they need. Depending on the amount of iron in your diet and the amount of iron in your prenatal vitamin-mineral supplement, you may not need to take additional iron. That's something that you can discuss with your healthcare provider, who will make recommendations based on the iron levels in your blood and your food choices.

Vegan Iron Sources

Even if you are taking an iron pill or getting most of the iron you need from your prenatal supplement, it still makes sense to choose foods high in iron. Why? These foods aren't just iron powerhouses; many of them are the basis for a healthy vegan diet because they are such good sources of other nutrients.

> Some foods have extra iron added. Two that come to mind are some brands of breakfast cereals and some veggie "meats." If you're looking for high-iron foods, check the Nutrition Facts label. If iron is added, you'll see larger numbers like 30 percent, 60 percent, or 100 percent in the iron row.

You've heard of some of these foods in earlier chapters—whole grains, dried beans, soy products, leafy green vegetables. Others may be less familiar. Did you know that a tablespoon of blackstrap molasses has more iron than ½ cup of spinach? Sea vegetables are another, possibly less familiar, iron source.

Making Good Choices: Breads and Cereals

Whole grains—foods like whole-wheat flour, brown rice, and oatmeal—have undergone minimal processing. These foods and other whole grains are good sources of iron. When grains are refined (think white flour, white rice, and degermed cornmeal), the part of the grain that contains the most iron is removed. Sure, this improves shelf life and, if you like the color white, makes for a more attractive product, but it also reduces the nutritional quality of the grain. In order to compensate for this, refined grains often have some nutrients added back, including iron. This means that both whole grains and enriched grains (refined grains that have some nutrients added back) are good sources of iron.

Another wonderful grain source of iron is wheat germ. Wheat germ is the high-iron part of wheat that is removed when wheat is refined. By adding a spoonful or two of wheat germ to smoothies or hot cereal, you can boost the iron in these foods.

Making Good Choices: Beans and Soy Foods

Dried beans and soy products are foods vegans turn to in order to meet their iron needs. A cup of cooked lentils has about as much iron as five and a half chicken drumsticks or a 9-ounce hamburger. All dried beans and peas are good sources of iron. Green beans, of course, are not dried beans and don't have the iron that dried beans do.

Some great vegan sources of iron don't fit neatly into categories like dried beans, vegetables, grains, or fruits. Foods like blackstrap molasses, dark chocolate, and energy bars are easy ways to add some extra iron. Blackstrap molasses is a by-product of sugar production. It is high not just in iron but also in calcium and other minerals.

Soy foods, based on soybeans, are also high in iron. Soybeans have more iron than other dried beans, so products made from soybeans like tofu, tempeh, and soy milk are also good sources of iron. Some veggie "meats" have extra iron added to them. Check the Nutrition Facts label to help identify these products.

Making Good Choices: Vegetables and Sea Vegetables

Vegetables vary widely in terms of their iron content. For instance, you'd have to eat 3½ cups of iceberg lettuce in order to get as much iron as you would from a single cup of raw spinach. Six cups of cooked cauliflower or carrot sticks would have as much iron as 1 cup of green peas. And it would take a whopping 8 cups of sautéed mushrooms to have as much iron as 1 cup of cooked collard greens.

As a group, green vegetables are good iron sources. Green vegetables include leafy greens like spinach, beet greens, collards, kale, and Swiss chard. Other green vegetables like asparagus, Brussels sprouts, and bok choy also contain iron. Tomato products, including sun-dried tomatoes, tomato juice, and tomato sauce, are another way to add iron to your diet.

Sea vegetables, as the name suggests, are vegetables harvested from the sea. You may have tried nori, a sea vegetable that forms the wrapping for sushi rolls. Other sea vegetables include kombu, dulse, and wakame (pronounced *wah-ka-may*). Sea vegetables are often sold in dried form and may need to be rehydrated before using. They have a pleasant, salty-sweet taste and can be added to salads, soups, grain dishes, or stir-fries. Kombu is especially high in iron, but most sea vegetables are also excellent sources of iron and other minerals.

Making Good Choices: Fruits and Nuts

If you're looking to fruit as a way to boost your iron intake, focus on dried fruits. Dried apricots, raisins, and prunes are actually not higher in iron than their fresh counterparts; it's just that most people can eat a handful of raisins without feeling as full as they would from eating an equivalent amount of grapes. Don't forget prune juice and apricot nectar—they're also ways to add iron.

> Roasted pumpkin seeds can be made at home using seeds from your Halloween jack-o'-lantern. Clean the seeds, removing all pumpkin flesh and strings. Let dry. Toss with a little oil, salt, and spices. Spread in a single layer on a cookie sheet and bake at 275°F for 10–20 minutes, checking often so they don't burn.

The best iron choices from the nuts and seeds food group are cashews, pumpkin seeds, and sunflower seeds. While other nuts do supply some iron, cashews have more iron than almonds, pecans, or walnuts.

Tahini (sesame seed butter) may be familiar if you're used to making your own hummus (it's an ingredient in many recipes). It can also be stirred into grains or vegetable dishes. With close to 3 milligrams of iron in 2 tablespoons, tahini has more iron than other nut or seed butters.

Top Vegan Iron Sources

While many foods vegans eat supply iron, the following foods are some of the highest sources:

1. Iron-fortified breakfast cereals (up to 18 milligrams in 1 ounce)
2. Cream of Wheat or instant oatmeal (up to 12 milligrams in 1 cup of prepared cereal)
3. Tofu (6.6 milligrams in ½ cup)
4. Kombu (1.1 milligrams in ¼ cup)
5. Iron-fortified energy bars (up to 2.7 milligrams in a bar)
6. Soybeans (4.5 milligrams in 1 cup)
7. Dark chocolate (1.8 milligrams in 1 ounce)
8. Lentils (6.6 milligrams in 1 cup)
9. Spinach (6.4 milligrams in 1 cup cooked)
10. Chickpeas (4.7 milligrams in 1 cup)

Menu Makeovers

One of the best things you can do during pregnancy is take some of your favorite vegan meals and see what changes you can make to boost their iron content. You'll probably find that you're eating healthier overall when you make these changes. For example, if your go-to breakfast is orange juice, Shredded Wheat with strawberries and soy milk, and toast with peanut butter, try these changes:

- Swirl some prune juice in with your OJ.
- Sprinkle a spoonful of wheat germ on your cereal along with the strawberries.
- Choose a higher-iron cereal—either a fortified ready-to-eat cereal or oatmeal.
- Try replacing the peanut butter with high-iron tahini and top your toast with raisins.

If you usually snack on pretzels and fruit, make an iron-rich trail mix with dried apricots, cashews, and pumpkin or sunflower seeds.

Here's a dinner makeover. If your menu features stir-fried green beans, broccoli, and carrots with almonds over brown rice:

- Replace all or part of the vegetables with higher-iron choices—peas, spinach, Swiss chard, for instance.
- Season the stir-fry with nori flakes.
- Add a higher-iron protein source like firm tofu cubes or some navy beans or other beans.
- In place of adding beans to the stir-fry, add another dish containing beans—maybe a hummus dip or lentil soup as an appetizer.
- Choose another grain, quinoa for example, or serve the stir-fry over enriched pasta.
- Treat yourself to a small piece of dark chocolate for dessert.

Making the Most of Dietary Iron

Nonheme iron, the only form of iron found in plants, is absorbed to a greater or lesser extent depending on the other foods that are eaten along with plant sources of iron. Substances called *phytates* are major inhibitors of iron absorption. Phytates are found in a number of foods vegans commonly eat, including whole grains, dried beans, nuts, seeds, and vegetables. It may seem that almost every food that you think of as a good vegan iron source contains these substances that interfere with iron absorption.

The good news is that foods that provide vitamin C can pretty much counter-act phytates' interfering actions. Something as simple as drinking a small glass of orange juice with a meal can increase the amount of iron that is absorbed by as much as 400 percent, even if phytates are present.

It's not just orange juice that can help increase iron absorption. All citrus fruits and juices provide vitamin C. So do tomatoes and tomato products (tomato sauce, tomato juice, and tomato soup), broccoli, cauliflower, cabbage, cantaloupe, kiwi, pineapple, kale, sweet potatoes—most fruits and many vegetables can add vitamin C.

The trick is to have the food that provides vitamin C at the same meal as the foods high in iron. For simplicity's sake, try to have a vitamin C source at most meals—a piece of fruit, a small glass of juice, or a serving of vegetables; not only will iron absorption be improved, but you'll also be eating healthier.

Another trick for promoting iron absorption is to use more foods produced or preserved by the action of microorganisms, commonly called *fermented foods*. These foods like sauerkraut, traditional soy sauce, tempeh, and sourdough bread contain organic acids that promote iron absorption.

Coffee (both regular and decaffeinated), tea (including some herb teas), and cocoa contain substances that interfere with iron absorption. If you use these beverages, wait to have them until several hours have gone by after a meal with a lot of iron in it to keep substances in the beverages from blocking your body's uptake of that iron.

Calcium supplements can also interfere with iron absorption. If you're taking calcium pills, take them between meals to be safe.

Iron Deficiency

About half of all pregnant women develop iron-deficiency anemia. That's because pregnant women need 1.5 times as much iron as they usually do when not pregnant, and because many women aren't getting enough iron even before they are pregnant. In fact, women frequently have low amounts of iron stored in their bodies.

There's no evidence that vegan women have higher rates of iron deficiency. Because iron-deficiency anemia can increase the risk of having a premature or low-birth-weight baby, it's routine to check the iron status of all pregnant women.

Anemia can make you feel weak, tired, and dizzy. So can pregnancy. A blood test is needed to help sort things out. Iron status is commonly checked by drawing a blood sample and determining the levels of hemoglobin and hematocrit. This is typically done at your first prenatal visit. Iron status may be checked again in the second and third trimesters, and it may be checked more frequently if your blood is low in iron.

If low levels are found, you will probably be given iron supplements to take. Additional tests of iron status may also need to be done. One such test is measuring blood levels of a substance called *ferritin*, which provides an indication of how much iron you have stored in your body. Ideally, you would have some extra iron stored to replace any blood losses or to compensate for times when you're not eating a lot of high-iron foods. It's not unusual for vegan and vegetarian women to have lower levels of ferritin even if their hematocrit and hemoglobin are in the normal range.

> Large doses of iron can be toxic. Take only the amount of iron recommended by your healthcare provider. Store iron supplements out of the reach of children and make sure that your bottle has a childproof cap if there are children in the house.

Iron-deficiency anemia can lead to pica—craving nonfood items such as clay, dirt, paper, or laundry starch, as well as ice, flour, or cornstarch. If you experience these types of cravings, let your healthcare provider know immediately. Nonfood items can contain toxins or contaminants that could be harmful to you and your baby and can interfere with nutrient absorption.

Supplement Strategy

In order to make sure you're getting enough iron, your healthcare provider will recommend an iron-enriched prenatal vitamin-mineral supplement, an iron supplement, or both. The level of iron you need will depend on your iron status. For example, the CDC recommends an iron supplement of 30 milligrams per day beginning at your first prenatal visit. If you're diagnosed with iron deficiency, a higher-dose supplement, 60–120 milligrams, may be prescribed. Talk to your healthcare provider to determine how much iron is right for you.

It's best to take iron supplements between meals or with a source of vitamin C (a glass of juice, for instance) to help your body absorb iron. If morning sickness is making it difficult to keep between-meal iron supplements down, temporarily try taking them with a meal.

Some women find that iron supplements, especially higher-dose supplements, lead to constipation. This may not affect you; vegan diets are typically quite high in fiber, so constipation is not something many vegans experience. If your iron supplements do seem to be constipating, try a daily glass of prune juice. Not only will this help make things move, but it's also a good way to add some iron. Making sure you're eating plenty of high-fiber foods like dried beans, whole grains, fruits, and vegetables can also help with constipation.

If you're taking an iron supplement, don't be concerned if you notice that your stools look darker than usual. This is a common side effect of high doses of iron and is not harmful. Of course, if you see blood in your stools, you should contact your healthcare provider right away.

High-dose iron supplements can interfere with the absorption of other minerals. If you're taking a higher dose of iron, your healthcare provider may check to make sure you're getting enough zinc and copper.

Vegan Zinc Sources

Zinc plays an important role in your baby's development. Luckily, many foods that are good sources of iron are also good sources of zinc, and prenatal supplements also typically contain zinc. Zinc deficiencies are rare in the United States. Mild zinc deficiencies may lead to poor appetite, a reduced sense of taste, and slower wound healing.

Zinc requirements go up with pregnancy, just like iron. Coincidentally, the amount of zinc that you absorb from meals increases also. Just as with iron, however, phytates and other substances in foods from plants can interfere with zinc absorption. As with iron, there are strategies that you can use to make the most of food sources of zinc.

An easy meal that provides almost half of the zinc recommendation for pregnancy consists of ¾ cup of curried chickpeas, 1½ cups of quinoa, and ½ cup of sautéed mushrooms. Add a sprinkling of chopped cashews to supply even more zinc. Key zinc sources in this meal are the chickpeas, quinoa, and mushrooms. Dried beans, whole grains, and zinc-fortified foods are all excellent zinc choices for vegans.

Some breakfast cereals are fortified with zinc, as are some veggie "meats" and energy bars. If you're looking for brands with higher zinc amounts, check the Nutrition Facts label at the grocery store. Just as it does with iron, adding a spoonful or two of wheat germ to hot cereals or other grain dishes adds extra zinc.

Vegetables that have the highest amounts of zinc include mushrooms, spinach, peas, corn, and asparagus. Fruits are not an especially good way to get zinc. Dark chocolate is not just a good way to get iron; it also provides zinc—and has more of either of these minerals than milk chocolate.

The following vegan foods are especially good zinc sources:

- Zinc-fortified breakfast cereals (up to 15 milligrams of zinc in 1 ounce of cereal)
- Wheat germ (2.7 milligrams in 2 tablespoons)
- Zinc-fortified veggie "meats" (up to 1.8 milligrams in 1 ounce)
- Zinc-fortified energy bars (up to 5.2 milligrams in a bar)
- Adzuki beans (4 milligrams in 1 cup)
- Tahini (1.4 milligrams in 2 tablespoons)
- Chickpeas (2.4 milligrams in 1 cup)
- Black-eyed peas (2.2 milligrams in 1 cup)
- Lentils (2.6 milligrams in 1 cup)
- Peanuts, peanut butter (close to 2 milligrams in 2 tablespoons)

Making the Most of Zinc

While zinc absorption is lower from beans and grains than it is from meats, there are definitely techniques that you can use to raise the amount of zinc you absorb from a vegan diet. Zinc is better absorbed from yeast-raised breads than from quick breads or muffins that are leavened with baking powder or baking soda. That doesn't mean that you can't eat quick breads or muffins; just be aware that yeast-raised breads provide more zinc. Zinc absorption is higher from fermented foods like sauerkraut, soy sauce, and tempeh. If you are into sprouting, you're in luck. Sprouting grains and beans reduces their phytate content and makes it easier to absorb the zinc in these foods.

These ideas are all ways to fine-tune your dietary zinc levels. If you don't have time to bake your own bread or sprout lentils, don't worry. Just check your prenatal supplement to make sure that it supplies zinc and take it regularly.

Chapter 5

Calcium and Vitamin D for Healthy Bones

Calcium and vitamin D are important nutrients for building strong bones and teeth when you are pregnant and when you aren't. Both of these nutrients can definitely be supplied by a vegan diet. For example, especially good sources of calcium include leafy greens—think kale and bok choy. Vitamin D is added to foods and is made by your body after you've been in the sun. Many nondairy milks are fortified with both calcium and vitamin D in forms that are easily absorbed. Your body even provides extra help—you absorb more calcium when you're pregnant.

Key Nutrients for Bone Health

Together, calcium and vitamin D are thought of as the most important nutrients for healthy bones, but other vitamins and minerals, along with protein, are also needed for bone health. When bones first develop, protein forms a sort of scaffolding that is filled in with the minerals calcium and phosphorus. Calcium and phosphorus are what make bones hard and unlikely to break. Vitamin D plays an important role because it increases the amount of calcium that is absorbed. Your bones need a constant supply of calcium because they are always changing and rebuilding, even when you're no longer growing. And, of course, when you're pregnant, you need calcium to form your baby's bones.

Other important nutrients for healthy bones include phosphorus, vitamin K, vitamin B_{12}, riboflavin, protein, and vitamin B_6. In other words, eating a well-balanced diet is one of the best things you can do to make sure that your bones get the nutrients they need.

Besides its important role in building strong bones, calcium is also important for building strong teeth. Even though your baby's teeth won't appear until sometime in the first year after birth, they're developing during pregnancy. Calcium also helps make baby's jawbone strong.

And it's not just nutrition that's important for bones. Exercise, especially weight-bearing exercise, such as walking, running, low-impact aerobics, or step aerobics, is important throughout your life to make sure that your bones stay strong as you get older. Exercise while pregnant won't really help your baby's bones, but it has other benefits.

Baby's Bone Development

Your baby's skeleton begins to develop in the third week after conception. Cool, right? Twenty-four weeks later, the bones are fully developed. That's a pretty quick turnaround. At this point, baby's bones are not hard like mature bones are; they are still soft and bend easily. By the time your baby is born, she'll have accumulated close to an ounce of calcium, most of it in her bones, all supplied by you. Your baby's bones will continue to mature after birth and will become harder and longer with time. Some bones will fuse together as the baby develops, so the total number of bones in adulthood is less than the number at birth.

Calcium Needs

Throughout your pregnancy, you will be meeting your baby's calcium needs. The calcium from foods you eat will move from your intestines, into your blood, through the placenta, and to your baby. Although your baby's bones are growing throughout pregnancy, the last trimester is peak growth time. During that trimester, he'll need 200–250 milligrams of calcium a day—a little less than the amount of calcium in a cup of fortified soy milk (if you absorbed all of that calcium). Since you absorb only a third or less of dietary calcium, the RDA for calcium is higher than 200–250 milligrams.

With pregnancy, calcium needs are higher in order to maintain your bones and to supply calcium for your baby's bone and teeth development. Remarkably, your body compensates for the increased calcium needs by pumping up the amount of calcium that you absorb from your food. Early in pregnancy, the amount of calcium you absorb doubles; higher calcium absorption continues throughout your pregnancy. Since calcium absorption is so high in pregnancy, the recommendation for how much calcium you need doesn't increase above what it was prepregnancy. So if you were getting the amount of calcium that you needed before you were pregnant and you're eating similar foods now, chances are good that you're meeting your calcium needs.

Vegan Calcium Sources

What's great is that almost every one of the food groups in a vegan's diet has foods that can markedly add to calcium intake. Calcium from nuts and seeds, vegetables, fruits, fruit juices, beans, and grains is very well absorbed. Typically, about 30 percent of the calcium in dairy products is absorbed. That same 30 percent is absorbed from foods fortified with calcium. Green vegetables are the true prizewinners when it comes to calcium; more than half of the calcium in green vegetables like kale, broccoli, and Chinese cabbage is absorbed.

Vegetables Provide Calcium

With a few exceptions, if a vegetable is green and has leaves, it is a good source of calcium. Calcium-rich vegetables include bok choy, broccoli, Chinese cabbage, collard greens, kale, mustard greens, and turnip greens. Even some nonleafy vegetables, including okra and butternut squash, supply some calcium. Calcium is added to some commercial vegetable juices also—check the Nutrition Facts label for calcium.

> A few foods contain oxalic acid, a substance that can interfere with calcium absorption from those foods. While food charts make spinach, Swiss chard, beet greens, rhubarb, and sweet potatoes look like good sources of calcium, the oxalic acid in these foods keeps you from absorbing much calcium from them.

You could get close to the calcium RDA of 1,000 milligrams by eating about 4–5 cups of cooked kale, collards, or turnip greens, and for someone who really loves greens, that is not impossible. Assuming you'd prefer to rely on some other foods also, it's still possible to get a generous dose of calcium from green vegetables without eating several bowls of them a day. You can add finely chopped greens to soups, chilis, stews, curries, pasta sauces, grains (green rice, anyone?), and mashed potatoes. Try sautéing chopped greens in a little olive oil and seasoning them with garlic and lemon juice. Add greens to stir-fries. Mild, tender greens like kale can be finely shredded and added to tossed salads or used in place of lettuce on burritos or wraps. Your options are endless!

Beans and Soy Foods Supply Calcium Too

Dried beans are another calcium source for vegans. Soybeans, black beans, great northern beans, and navy beans are especially high in calcium. Other dried beans, while not superstars, can still add to your calcium intake.

Since soybeans are high in calcium, foods made from soybeans also supply calcium. Tempeh, soy nuts (roasted soybeans), TVP, and tofu are all naturally rich calcium sources. Tofu is made by mixing soy milk with a mineral salt to make the soy milk firm up (sort of like making cheese). Many tofu makers use nigari (magnesium chloride) as a coagulating agent. Calcium sulfate is another coagulating agent that is also used. Tofu made with calcium sulfate is especially high in calcium; however, if you can only find tofu made with nigari, you are still getting some calcium from the soybeans that were used to make the tofu.

> If you're relying on calcium-fortified soy milk or other plant milks as one of your calcium mainstays, be sure to shake the milk thoroughly before pouring it. That will help to make sure that the calcium is mixed in and doesn't settle to the bottom of the carton.

If you purchase calcium-fortified soy milk, you'll be buying soy milk that has calcium added to it. This calcium is well absorbed. Many brands of soy milk supply as much calcium per cup as cow's milk. Check the label of your favorite brand to make sure calcium has been added. Some brands of vegan cheese and yogurt are also fortified with calcium.

Don't Forget Nuts, Seeds, Fruits, Grains, and Other Foods

While greens, tofu, and calcium-fortified soy milk can supply enough calcium to meet your needs, there are many other foods that are either naturally high in calcium or that are fortified with calcium.

Almond butter, sesame seeds, and tahini are the best sources of calcium when it comes to nuts and seeds. Fruits are not especially high in calcium with the exception of figs—a cup of dried figs has almost as much calcium as a cup of collard greens. Dried figs can also help with the constipation that can be a feature in late pregnancy. Try eating a few figs for snacks or adding them to hot cereal.

If you look in your supermarket's refrigerated or frozen section, you'll see that many brands of juice, especially orange juice, are calcium-fortified. If you're trying to increase your calcium, choosing a fortified juice is an easy way to do it.

Many commercial breakfast cereals are fortified with calcium. The Nutrition Facts label can help you decide which cereals are good calcium sources—look for 300 milligrams or more of calcium in a serving. Plant milks like rice milk, almond milk, and oat milk are also often fortified with calcium.

Adding a spoonful of blackstrap molasses to hot cereals, muffin batter, baked beans, or stews is another way to boost your calcium intake. A tablespoon of blackstrap molasses provides 200 milligrams of calcium.

While many foods vegans eat supply calcium, the following foods are some of the highest sources:

- Calcium-fortified plant milks (up to 450 milligrams in 1 cup)
- Dried figs (120 milligrams in ½ cup)
- Tofu (especially prepared with calcium sulfate) (up to 434 milligrams in 4 ounces)
- Collard greens (268 milligrams in 1 cup cooked greens)
- Kale (177 milligrams in 1 cup cooked greens)
- Turnip greens (197 milligrams in 1 cup cooked greens)
- Bok choy (158 milligrams in 1 cup cooked greens)
- Calcium-fortified orange juice (350 milligrams in 1 cup)
- Blackstrap molasses (400 milligrams in 2 tablespoons)
- Soybeans (175 milligrams in 1 cup)
- Navy beans (126 milligrams in 1 cup)

Calcium Supplements

Many prenatal vitamin-mineral supplements do not supply much calcium. Check the label of the brand that you are using. Ideally, you would be getting the calcium you need from foods. If your diet is low in calcium, however, and your prenatal supplement has little or no calcium, a separate calcium supplement may be needed. The two most common forms of calcium supplements are calcium carbonate and calcium citrate. Each kind has some advantages.

Calcium carbonate is usually less expensive, and fewer tablets may be needed. It is absorbed best when taken with food. The drawback of taking calcium supplements with foods is that the calcium interferes with iron absorption.

Calcium supplements made with calcium citrate can be taken between meals, so there's less chance that they'll interfere with iron absorption. In addition, they do not need stomach acid to be absorbed. If you are on acid-blocking medications such as omeprazole (Prilosec), this is the preferable form of calcium for you to take.

Calcium supplements may cause you to have more gas or to feel bloated or constipated. If that happens, try to take several smaller doses of calcium supplements throughout the day or try a different brand.

Myths and Facts about Calcium

One of the simplest myths about calcium is that you need to consume dairy products to get enough calcium in your diet. Look around at plant-eating animals like horses and cows—their massive bones are all made from calcium from plant foods. Milk is not a part of their adult diet.

Protein and Calcium

The relationship among protein, calcium, and bone health is a complex one. Older research suggested that people on very high-protein diets had a lot of calcium in their urine. In other words, they were losing calcium rather than storing it. This research led to the idea that people whose diets were lower in protein lost less calcium. Since their calcium losses were lower, the theory was that people on lower-protein diets would not need as much calcium. Some vegans seized on this idea and guessed that vegans wouldn't need as much calcium as meat eaters do since the vegan diet is typically lower in protein.

Very high intakes of calcium have been associated with kidney stones, not something anyone wants. It's unlikely you'll go over the safe upper limit for calcium of 2,500 milligrams a day from your diet, but if you're also taking calcium supplements, it can happen. Check the labels of all supplements for their calcium content.

More recent studies have found that both adequate protein and adequate calcium are needed to produce strong bones less likely to fracture. Vegans should try to meet the RDA for calcium and to have enough protein in their diets.

Vitamin D: The Sunshine Vitamin

Vitamin D is known as the "sunshine vitamin" because your body makes vitamin D when your skin is exposed to the sun. Vitamin D is needed for your body to absorb calcium, so it is often linked to healthy bones. Only a few foods contain vitamin D naturally—mushrooms are one example of a vegan food that provides some vitamin D. Some mushrooms that have recently become available are exposed to ultraviolet light, which increases their vitamin D content. The main dietary source of vitamin D for many Americans is the vitamin D added to cow's milk. Vegan sources of vitamin D are also fortified foods; vitamin D is added to some brands of plant milks, fruit juices, and breakfast cereals.

Vitamin D needs do not increase in pregnancy. The RDA for vitamin D in pregnancy is 600 IU, the same as for nonpregnant women.

Vitamin D Production

It doesn't take much sun exposure to make all the vitamin D that you need. If you're fair skinned and can be out in the summer sun, experts estimate that you need about five to ten minutes a few times a week on your arms and face to meet your needs. This is a very rough estimate, however, and many factors can affect the production of vitamin D.

Sunscreen and clothing block vitamin D production, so if you'd like to get vitamin D from the sun, wait a few minutes before putting on sunscreen or covering up. Remember though, that use of sunscreen is important to lower your risk for skin cancer, so never skip it altogether.

If your skin is darker or if you live where there's a lot of air pollution or it's a cloudy day, you will need more sun exposure to make vitamin D. Winter sun in the northern part of the United States is not strong enough to promote vitamin D production. If you live in the north in the winter, don't get out in the sun that much, or use sunscreen or protective clothing whenever you're outside, you'll need to know about other ways to meet your vitamin D needs.

Your body produces only the vitamin D that it needs, so even with a large dose of sunlight you won't make excessive amounts of vitamin D. Of course, too much sun has potential to increase your risk of skin cancer, so don't overdo it!

Vitamin D Sources for Vegans

Look to fortified foods and supplements for most of your vitamin D. Vitamin D is added to many brands of plant milks, including almond milk, hemp milk, coconut milk, rice milk, and soy milk. Some brands of dairy look-alikes (like yogurt and cheese) also have vitamin D added. Breakfast cereals, juices, and energy bars are some other products often fortified with vitamin D.

Fresh mushrooms that are identified on the label as being a good source of vitamin D have been exposed to ultraviolet light that stimulated the mushroom's production of vitamin D. A 3-ounce serving of these mushrooms has about 400 IU of vitamin D, about two-thirds of the recommended daily intake.

Vitamin D supplements are another option. Many calcium supplements also contain vitamin D and so do most prenatal supplements. Before taking extra vitamin D (beyond what is in your prenatal supplement), check with your healthcare provider or RD to make sure you're not overdoing this vitamin.

Vitamin D_2 versus Vitamin D_3

Vitamin D is found in two different forms in supplements and fortified foods. Vitamin D_2, also called *ergocalciferol*, is made from yeast exposed to ultraviolet light. Vitamin D_2 is a vegan form of vitamin D. Vitamin D_3, also called *cholecalciferol*, is often made from lanolin from sheep's wool and, if it is from wool, is not considered vegan. A vegan form of vitamin D_3 is made from lichen and is available in supplement form. Both forms of vitamin D are effective ways to meet requirements.

Most, although not all, brands of soy milk and other plant milks are fortified with vitamin D_2. Breakfast cereals, orange juice, and margarine are commonly fortified with nonvegan vitamin D_3. High–vitamin D mushrooms contain vitamin D_2; supplements may contain either D_2 or D_3. If you would prefer to avoid nonvegan vitamin D_3, check the ingredient listing on products that you use. Most products will identify either vitamin D_3 or vitamin D_2 in the list of ingredients; if vitamin D_3 is the vegan form, it will be identified as such. If a package simply says vitamin D, you can contact the company to ask about the kind of vitamin D added to that product.

Chapter 6

Vitamin B, Folic Acid, DHA, and Iodine

Some of the most exciting times for a mom are when her baby first makes eye contact, smiles, and begins to talk. It's as if you can see your baby's brain growing as one new skill after another is acquired. Just like all of baby's systems, the nervous system (including the brain and nerves) develops rapidly before birth and in the weeks and months after birth. Vitamin B_{12}, folic acid, DHA, and iodine are all nutrients that, along with protein, are needed to build a healthy nervous system.

Vitamin B_{12} Is Essential for Vegans

Although only a very small amount (less than a gram) of vitamin B_{12} is needed, it is essential for health. Having one or more daily, reliable sources of vitamin B_{12} is especially important when you're not only providing for yourself but also responsible for meeting the needs of your unborn, and later (if you're breastfeeding) newborn, baby. Vitamin B_{12} stored in your body may not be available for transportation through the placenta or in breast milk to your baby, but vitamin B_{12} from diet or supplements is. That's why it's important to get this vitamin every day from food or supplements.

Vitamin B_{12} plays an important role in developing and maintaining the nervous system. Deficiencies of this nutrient are rare, but when they occur, they can have serious consequences, including developmental delays, difficulty walking, and permanent damage to the nervous system. Vitamin B_{12} deficiency can cause issues in adults, but in pregnancy it is all about the baby and preventing both developmental problems as well as preterm labor.

In nature, all vitamin B_{12} is produced by microorganisms; neither animals nor plants can make the vitamin. Vitamin B_{12} is found in meat, milk, eggs, and other animal-based foods because animals eat microorganisms that contain it. There are no reliable plant-based sources of vitamin B_{12} other than foods fortified with it. The limited number of nonanimal sources of vitamin B_{12} makes it a nutrient vegans have to pay attention to. Getting enough as a vegan is an easy issue to address, but one that is important to be proactive about.

Vegan Sources of Vitamin B_{12}

Fortunately for vegans, many food manufacturers add vitamin B_{12} to their products—check labels to see if vitamin B_{12} is added to foods you use. Some vegan products that commonly (or at least sometimes) have vitamin B_{12} added are:

- Plant milks
- Energy bars and protein bars
- Marmite yeast extract
- Tofu

- Nutritional yeast
- Veggie "meats"
- Breakfast cereals

Companies have been known to change their product formulation, especially with regard to vitamin fortification. Check the label of foods you rely on for vitamin B_{12} frequently so you're not lulled into thinking a product has vitamin B_{12} when it no longer does.

Nutritional Yeast

Nutritional yeast, a mild-tasting, light-yellow flake or powder, is a good source of vitamin B_{12} if the yeast is grown with a medium containing vitamin B_{12}. Nutritional yeast containing this vitamin is commonly available in packages and in bulk food bins. Check the label to make sure the product you are using contains it. A heaping tablespoon of Red Star Vegetarian Support Formula (VSF) Yeast Flakes (large flakes) supplies 4 micrograms of vitamin B_{12}.

Nutritional yeast is a versatile ingredient that can be added to many dishes. Here are some ideas:

- Sprinkle on freshly popped popcorn along with a bit of salt or chili powder
- Mix with bread crumbs and use to top a casserole or in breading
- Add to your favorite scrambled tofu recipe
- Use to add flavor to steamed vegetables, grain and pasta dishes, soups, vegan pizza, and other foods commonly topped with Parmesan cheese
- Mix in with mashed potatoes
- Mix in with bread dough to add a cheesy taste to breadsticks or other savory breads
- Use to top breakfast toast (along with vegan margarine)
- Make a nutritional yeast-based dip

Getting Enough Vitamin B_{12}

Most prenatal vitamins contain vitamin B_{12}. If your prenatal supplement supplies at least 2.6 micrograms of vitamin B_{12} and you take it daily in the amount recommended, you should be set. If your prenatal supplement doesn't supply it, you'll need to seek out other sources—a separate vitamin B_{12} supplement providing at least 2.6 micrograms (some vegan dietitians recommend as much as 25–100 micrograms). Talk to you doctor about what is right for you.

> Vitamin B_{12} comes in tablet and capsule form and also comes in drops and tablets that can be used under the tongue. Compounding pharmacies can make it into a nasal spray as well. (Vitamin B_{12} is often absorbed better by avoiding the stomach.)

While people may point out that very few vegans develop vitamin B_{12} deficiencies, it's much better to be safe than sorry!

Don't Count on These Foods for Vitamin B_{12}

Foods reported to contain vitamin B_{12} include fermented foods (tempeh, sauerkraut, miso, sourdough bread), umeboshi plums, sea vegetables, shiitake mushrooms, spirulina (algae), and soybeans. None of these—or any plant foods, for that matter—contain enough vitamin B_{12} to prevent a deficiency. In fact, some of these foods contain a vitamin B_{12} analogue (something that looks like vitamin B_{12} but isn't) that can interfere with the vitamin's absorption from other foods. Do your homework before putting these foods in your body.

Folic Acid for Vegans

Folic acid (folate) is another essential vitamin. It's especially important early in pregnancy when the baby's neural tube is being formed. The neural tube develops into the brain and the spinal cord (the central nervous system). Adequate intake of folic acid while the neural tube is formed reduces the risk of birth defects like spina bifida.

A typical vegan diet includes many foods that are good sources of folate, including dried beans, leafy vegetables, oranges, orange juice, and peanuts. Folic acid is in breads, cereals, rice, pasta, flour, and other grain products.

Because folic acid is so important, the CDC recommends that pregnant women take a vitamin or eat a fortified food (some breakfast cereals are fortified, for example) that contains at least 100 percent of the DV for folic acid every day, or a combination of both methods. In fact, because a woman may not be aware that she is pregnant at the time when the fetus's neural tube starts to form, the CDC's recommendations for folic acid apply to all women of childbearing age, not just pregnant women.

DHA's Role

Docosahexaenoic acid (DHA) is a fatty acid most commonly found in the oil from fish. However, vegans can get DHA without having to eat salmon, tuna, or other fish. DHA, categorized as an omega-3 fatty acid, plays a role in the development of your baby's vision. DHA may also affect your baby's cognitive development, as noted in a *Nutrients* journal article from 2016.

In the last trimester, the fetus stores DHA in her brain and in her retina (a part of the eye). If your diet is low in DHA, stored DHA from your body will be used to meet your fetus's needs. Some experts fear this will make your stores of DHA too low.

There is a great deal of interest in DHA, and many research studies are being conducted. Some studies have found that blood levels of DHA in pregnant vegetarians are lower than in pregnant nonvegetarians. Whether or not this makes any difference is not known. Researchers have also found that if the mother has a higher DHA intake in pregnancy, her infant's visual acuity at four months is improved, although this effect is not seen at age six months. Small improvements in developmental function are also seen in infants whose mothers had higher DHA intakes in pregnancy.

DHA Without Fish

When it comes to DHA, vegans can get some DHA indirectly by taking alpha-linolenic acid (ALA), another omega-3 fatty acid, which is converted to DHA. Additionally, vegans can get DHA by taking vegan DHA supplements.

Make Your Own DHA

ALA is another omega-3 fatty acid your body is able to use to make DHA. Rates of production are slow, however, so it is unlikely you can make all the DHA you need in pregnancy. Still, you can get some DHA by making your own.

Besides being a building block for DHA, ALA is important on its own, so even if you're not counting on it to make DHA, having good sources of ALA is a part of a healthy vegan diet. Foods that are especially high in ALA are flaxseeds, flaxseed oil, canola oil, hemp seeds, hemp seed oil, chia seeds, walnuts, and walnut oil.

Flaxseeds are small dark-brown seeds with a slightly nutty taste. You can find them in breakfast cereals, breads, and even snack crackers and tortilla chips. Whole flaxseeds add a nice crunch, but that's about all; the fact is that most of them pass through your body undigested because of their hull. In order to release the ALA from flaxseeds, the seeds need to be ground into flaxseed meal, a powder that can be used in baking or added to smoothies. You can grind your own using a spice or coffee grinder or purchase it already ground. Flaxseed meal should be stored in the refrigerator or freezer.

> Flaxseed oil is added to many foods. If you'd like to get more omega-3 fats, look for peanut butter or vegan margarine with added flaxseed oil. Of course, you can make your own flaxseed oil–enhanced peanut butter by mixing a spoonful of flaxseed oil with a couple spoonfuls of peanut butter.

Flaxseed oil can be added to foods after they have been cooked, but it should not be used for cooking—the heat destroys the healthy fats. It's fine to mix flaxseed oil with steamed vegetables, cooked pasta, hot cereals, or other warm foods. It can be used to make salad dressings and can be added to smoothies without altering their taste. Just like flaxseed meal, flaxseed oil should be stored in the refrigerator or freezer.

Hemp seeds and hemp seed oil come from the hemp plant. You may have noticed hemp seeds, hemp milk, hemp flour, hemp oil, and hemp butter as well as products with added hemp at the grocery store. Shelled hemp seeds can be sprinkled onto foods or used in baking. Hemp seed butter can be used in place of peanut butter, and hemp flour is a gluten-free product.

DHA from Microalgae

Some people think fish are a good source of DHA because fish make their own DHA. Wrong! Fish, like people, don't make DHA. Fish actually get DHA the same way vegans (and others who don't eat fish) do: by eating algae. Certain algae naturally contain DHA. The oil from these algae is used to make vegan DHA supplements and to fortify foods with nonfish DHA.

Besides being a good source of ALA, hemp seeds supply other essential nutrients. Two tablespoons of shelled hemp seeds have about 80 calories and supply as much protein as ½ cup of beans. That same amount of hemp seeds provides generous amounts of iron, folic acid, and zinc.

Expert groups, including the International Society for the Study of Fatty Acids and Lipids (ISSFAL) and the American Academy of Pediatrics, recommend an intake of 200 milligrams daily of DHA for pregnant and lactating women. The easiest way to get DHA is to take a DHA supplement.

If you are interested in finding foods with vegan DHA, check the ingredient listing for DHA microalgal oil. Not all foods that contain DHA microalgal oil are vegan; the oil is also added to some brands of cow's milk, yogurt, and other nonvegan products.

Some prenatal supplements contain vegan DHA. Again, check for microalgal oil on the ingredient list.

Iodine Is Important Also

Iodine, a mineral that you may have heard of because it is added to iodized salt, is essential for the development of your baby's brain. Worldwide, iodine deficiency in pregnancy and early childhood is the single most important preventable cause of brain damage. Iodine needs are higher in pregnancy to be sure your baby gets enough iodine for brain development.

Because of variations in soil iodine in the United States, in 1924, the government approved the addition of iodine to salt. To see if the salt you use is iodized, check the package. Commercial sea salt contains variable amounts of iodine; at least one brand has iodine added. Three-quarters of a teaspoon of iodized salt provides enough iodine to meet the RDA for pregnancy.

Many people don't use this much salt. If you don't or if you use sea salt or other noniodized salt, you may need an iodine supplement. Many prenatal supplements contain iodine, but not all do. The American Thyroid Association recommends that pregnant women take a daily prenatal vitamin that contains at least 150 micrograms of iodine. The best way to check the amount that is right for you is to speak to your healthcare provider. As always, when in doubt, ask!

Sea vegetables like nori and kombu can provide some iodine, but amounts are variable. Some sea vegetables are very high in iodine. Arame, hiziki, and kombu are examples of high-iodine sea vegetables, but because excess iodine can cause health problems for you and your baby, you should limit use of these high-iodine sea vegetables during pregnancy.

Chapter 7

Vitamins and Supplements

Fruits, vegetables, whole grains, nuts, and dried beans that are mainstays of vegan diets supply key vitamins and minerals to the body. Still, women's diets are often low in nutrients such as iron, zinc, magnesium, and vitamins E and D. Pregnancy is a great opportunity to evaluate and revise your dietary habits, if necessary. Morning sickness, lack of time, and other situations can sabotage your best intentions; prenatal and other dietary supplements can help ensure you're getting the nutrients you need.

Vitamins and Minerals in Pregnancy

In pregnancy, and later if breastfeeding, women need more calories, protein, and some vitamins and minerals to meet the needs of their growing baby. Most of these nutrients can come from your regular diet, but supplements may be needed for some nutrients that are commonly in short supply. The following table shows how recommendations for some vitamins and minerals change in pregnancy and during breastfeeding.

Recommended Dietary Allowance for Vegan Women Age 19–50 Years

Nutrient	Nonpregnant	Pregnant	Breastfeeding
Calcium	1,000 mg	1,000 mg	1,000 mg
Iodine	150 mcg	220 mcg	290 mcg
Magnesium	310 mg (19–30 years) 320 mg (31–50 years)	350 mg (19–30 years) 360 mg (31–50 years)	310 mg (19–30 years) 320 mg (31–50 years)
Iron	32 mg	49 mg	16 mg
Zinc	8 mg	11 mg	12 mg
Vitamin A	700 mcg	770 mcg	1,300 mcg
Vitamin D	15 mcg	15 mcg	15 mcg
Vitamin E	15 mg	15 mg	19 mg
Vitamin K (Adequate intake)	90 mcg	90 mcg	90 mcg
Thiamin	1.1 mg	1.4 mg	1.4 mg
Riboflavin	1.1 mg	1.4 mg	1.6 mg
Niacin	14 mg	18 mg	17 mg
Vitamin B_6	1.3 mg	1.9 mg	2.0 mg
Folate	400 mcg	600 mcg	500 mcg
Vitamin B_{12}	2.4 mcg	2.6 mcg	2.8 mcg
Vitamin C	75 mg	85 mg	120 mg

RDAs from the Food and Nutrition Board, Institute of Medicine, National Academies (Institute of Medicine is now known as the Health and Medicine Division).

Please note that because iron absorption from plant-derived foods is lower than from meat and fish, the Food and Nutrition Board, Institute of Medicine, National Academies (Institute of Medicine is now known as the Health and Medicine Division) calls for multiplying the iron RDA for nonvegetarians by a factor of 1.8. This new number is the RDA for iron for vegetarians. The iron RDAs in this table have been calculated based on the nonvegetarian RDA times 1.8.

Although recommendations are higher in pregnancy for magnesium, vitamin A, thiamin, riboflavin, niacin, vitamin B_6, and vitamin C, it's likely that as you increase the amount of food you eat, you'll also get more of these nutrients (assuming you're eating a reasonably healthy diet). The RDA for iron in pregnancy is challenging for most women to meet from diet alone. Zinc can also be difficult, especially if you're relying mainly on beans and grains as zinc sources. Folate and iodine supplements are recommended in pregnancy. Vegan women need to use either fortified foods or a supplement to meet vitamin B_{12} needs.

Women who are pregnant should not take regular vitamins; they could be too low in some nutrients and too high in others. Ask your healthcare provider about special prenatal supplements, which contain the vitamins and minerals you will need during your pregnancy. Be sure to tell your healthcare provider about any vitamins you are already taking before adding a prenatal vitamin supplement.

Choosing a Prenatal Vitamin–Mineral Supplement

Your healthcare provider may recommend a specific brand of prenatal vitamins because she likes the amounts and kinds of vitamins and minerals in it. You may opt to use this recommendation, but it may or may not be vegan. If taking a vegan prenatal supplement is important to you, discuss options with your healthcare provider. You can research brands and nutrients supplied by each product online and compare available vegan supplements to the supplement your provider recommends.

A good place to start researching what is available is on websites of companies that make vegan supplements. These include VegLife (www.nutraceutical.com/collections/healthy/veglife/), DEVA (www.devanutrition.com), Freeda Vitamins (https://freedavitamins.com), and Country Life (www.country-life.com). Websites of companies carrying vegan products can also be helpful. See Appendix A for some ideas.

If you are choosing a vegan prenatal supplement, you will need to be sure it meets your needs for essential nutrients low in your diet. A visit to an RD is one way to assess your diet. Expert groups, including the US Preventive Services Task Force and the American Thyroid Association, respectively, suggest that pregnant women take a 400–800 microgram folic acid supplement as well as a supplement providing 150 micrograms of iodine. Having a prenatal supplement that provides these nutrients reduces the number of pills you have to swallow. Other nutrients that can be challenging for vegans in pregnancy include iron, zinc, vitamin B_{12}, calcium, and vitamin D. If your diet doesn't meet your needs for these nutrients, look for a vegan prenatal supplement that can provide at least some of the amount needed and plan to get the rest from your food.

Share what you've learned with your provider and get his approval of any supplement you want to use. Be aware that prenatal supplements vary in terms of which nutrients and the amount of each nutrient that is included. For example, several brands of vegan prenatal supplements do not supply iodine, and the amount of zinc ranges from two-thirds to three times the zinc recommendation.

If you have questions about a specific supplement, including whether or not it is vegan, contact the manufacturer for more information.

Supplement Quality

Some independent organizations assess the quality of certain dietary supplements. They check to be sure the supplement contains what it says it does on the label. These quality certifications do not mean the product is safe or effective; the organizations assess only the manufacturing process. Supplement manufacturers are not required to participate in this type of evaluation program. Organizations that evaluate supplements include:

- ConsumerLab.com (www.consumerlab.com)
- NSF International (www.nsf.org)
- USP (www.usp.org)
- Natural Products Association TruLabel program (www.npanational.org)

Questions about the manufacturing process or possible contaminants can also be directed to supplement manufacturers.

Iron Supplements

Iron needs are high in pregnancy to support your increased blood volume and to stock iron stores for your baby. Add on the higher iron recommendations for vegetarians and vegans and it's virtually impossible to meet iron needs from diet alone, even with careful planning. You can refer to Chapter 4 for more information about iron.

Most pregnant women take some sort of iron supplement, either in their prenatal supplement or separately. Your provider will check your blood to assess your iron status. This information will help him determine how much supplemental iron you need to take.

> If your healthcare provider recommends you take supplemental iron, be sure to tell her about any medications you are using. Some drugs should not be taken with iron supplements.

Most prenatal supplements contain either 18 milligrams or 27 milligrams of iron. This, in conjunction with good dietary sources of iron, may be enough, or your provider may want you to take an additional low-dose iron supplement. If you're diagnosed with iron deficiency, a higher-dose supplement, 60–120 milligrams of iron, may be prescribed. Talk to your healthcare provider to determine how much iron is right for you.

Additional Supplements

In addition to a standard prenatal supplement and possibly iron, you may be wondering about additional supplements. Here is what several expert groups suggest. The US Preventive Services Task Force recommends that pregnant women get 400–800 micrograms daily of folic acid from supplements or fortified foods, or a combination of the two. The American Thyroid Association recommends that pregnant women take a prenatal vitamin that contains 150 micrograms of iodine every day—more can be obtained through other foods and iodized salt. The best way to check the amount that is right for you is to speak to your healthcare provider. As always, when in doubt, ask!

The RDA for vitamin B_{12} for pregnancy is 2.6 micrograms, which can come from supplements or fortified foods. If these nutrients in these amounts are not being supplied by your prenatal supplement (or by fortified foods, if that is an option), let your doctor know so that other sources can be explored.

If you need to take high-dose iron supplements, your healthcare provider may recommend a supplement of zinc and copper as well. Large amounts of iron can interfere with zinc and copper absorption.

Supplement Timing

Some supplements are better absorbed if they are taken with meals; some are better taken between meals. It can be a delicate balance. It's most important that you do take any necessary supplements, and that you and your doctor figure out the best timing to do so to improve the odds that you'll get the maximum benefit from the supplement.

Take iron supplements between meals to promote better absorption. Iron absorption can also be enhanced by taking your supplement with a vitamin C source such as orange juice or fresh tangerine juice. Remember that tea and coffee contain substances that can inhibit your absorption of iron (as well as calcium), so try to avoid using these to wash down supplements.

If you're suffering from morning sickness and find it difficult to keep your supplements down, you should try taking them with a meal. As your morning sickness improves, you can return to the between-meals dosing schedule.

If you are taking a calcium supplement, it should be taken separately from your iron supplement or from a prenatal supplement that contains iron. Calcium carbonate supplements are best absorbed with food.

The timing of other supplements—vitamin B_{12}, folic acid, DHA, iodine—is not that important. What is important is to regularly use any supplements recommended by your healthcare provider.

Too Much of a Good Thing — Avoiding Vitamin Excess

Vitamin and mineral supplements may seem like harmless pills. They are available without a prescription and may be something you take without much thought. In reality, taking too much of some vitamins and minerals can cause health problems. In pregnancy, excesses of some vitamins could be harmful to your baby. For example, very high levels of vitamin A have been linked to birth defects. The simplest way to avoid a problem is to take only the vitamins and minerals that have been approved by your doctor. Dietary supplements are meant to supplement your diet; they do not take the place of eating a healthy, varied vegan diet.

Herbal Supplements in Pregnancy

It's tempting to think that herbal and botanical supplements and remedies are universally safe to use in pregnancy. In reality, just because something seems to come from nature does not automatically guarantee it is safe. Think of poison ivy, mistletoe, and some mushrooms—all natural and all potentially dangerous. Even herbs that can be used when you're not pregnant can be harmful to your developing baby. Always check with your provider before taking any sort of supplement or remedy.

Some herbal remedies claim they will help with pregnancy. These claims may or may not be true or based on actual research. Herbal remedies and "natural products" do not have to be approved by the US Food and Drug Administration (FDA) for safety or truth in labeling. Makers of herbal remedies do not have to determine whether or not their products are safe to use in pregnancy, either. Scary, right?

The National Center for Complementary and Integrative Health (formerly the National Center for Complementary and Alternative Medicine) provides guidance on the use of some herbs in pregnancy. Following is a partial list of products to avoid in pregnancy:

- Products that contain bitter orange, black cohosh, and red clover should not be used due to a lack of safety evidence. These should also be avoided by nursing women.

- Ephedra, yohimbe, and goldenseal should be avoided in pregnancy and when breastfeeding.
- Cat's-claw should be avoided because of its use in the past to prevent pregnancy.
- Chasteberry can affect hormone levels.
- Fenugreek, feverfew, and licorice can induce premature delivery.

This is not an all-inclusive list of products to avoid. Before using any herbal or botanical product, consult your healthcare provider. In addition to affecting your baby's health, these products can also interfere with medications and have an effect on conditions like gestational diabetes and high blood pressure.

Part 3

Vegan Lifestyle

Chapter 8

Putting It All Together

You've heard it before—whole grains, beans, fruits, vegetables, and nuts are the basis for a healthy vegan diet. But maybe that's not enough. How many servings of vegetables should you be eating now that you're pregnant? Are there foods that you should avoid? A simple vegan food guide for pregnancy can help. And if you'd like even more support, a session with a knowledgeable RD is a very worthwhile undertaking.

Vegan Food Guide for Pregnancy

Many food guides don't work for vegans. Food guides often include a meat group and a dairy group. Even if you replace meat with vegetable protein sources, you're still left with a food group that recommends eating cheese and drinking cow's milk.

This Vegan Food Guide for Pregnancy is based on five food groups. All servings listed are the minimum number of servings from each food group. If you are not gaining weight at the recommended rate, you'll need to eat a larger number of servings from the food groups. Be sure to choose a variety of foods from each food group.

Vegan Food Guide for Pregnancy

Food Group	Daily Servings
Grains	6
Dried Beans, Nuts, Milks, and Other Protein-Rich Foods	7
Vegetables	4
Fruits	2
Fats	2

In addition to making food choices based on this food guide, you should also be taking a prenatal supplement that supplies vitamins and minerals, including iron, zinc, iodine, vitamin B_{12}, and vitamin D. Supplemental DHA is also recommended in pregnancy. See previous chapters for more information on supplements.

Grains Group

This group includes breads, tortillas, crackers, bagels, rolls, pastas, rices, cereals, quinoa, and other foods made from grains. Choose whole grains as often as possible. A serving from this group is a slice of bread; a tortilla or roll; ½ cup of cooked cereal, grain, or pasta; or 1 ounce of ready-to-eat cereal. This food group provides carbohydrates, calories, fiber, B vitamins, iron, and some protein. Fortified cereals can supply other vitamins and minerals.

Dried Beans, Nuts, Milks, and Other Protein-Rich Foods Group

This food group includes a variety of foods that are good sources of protein for vegans. Many foods in this group also supply iron and zinc, and some foods are fortified with calcium, vitamin D, and vitamin B_{12}. A serving from this group is ½ cup of cooked dried beans or peas; ½ cup of tofu, TVP, or tempeh; 1 ounce of veggie "meat"; 2 tablespoons of nut or seed butters; ¼ cup of nuts or soy nuts; or 1 cup of fortified soy milk.

> The Vegan Food Guide for Pregnancy can also be used when you are breastfeeding. For most food groups, eat the same amounts as you did when you were pregnant. Choose one more serving of protein-rich foods, continue to use prenatal vitamins, and add foods as needed to prevent excess weight loss.

Vegetables Group

This food group includes all vegetables, from asparagus to zucchini. Vegetables can be eaten raw or cooked. A serving from this group is ½ cup of cooked vegetables or 1 cup of raw vegetables. Be sure to include some nutrient-rich dark-green vegetables and deep-orange vegetables often. This food group is an especially good source of fiber and vitamins A and C; it supplies some iron and zinc.

Fruits Group

Fruits are especially good sources of vitamins C and A; they also provide fiber and B vitamins. This group includes fresh, frozen, canned, and dried fruits and fruit juices. A serving from this group is a piece of medium fruit; ½ cup of cut-up or canned fruit; ¼ cup of dried fruit; or ½ cup of fruit juice.

Fats Group

This group provides calories, vitamin E, and essential fatty acids. Foods in this group include oils, vegan salad dressings and mayonnaise, vegan margarine, and vegan cream cheese. A serving of any of these foods is 1 teaspoon.

Meeting Calcium Needs with the Vegan Food Guide for Pregnancy

Vegans get calcium from different food groups. Green leafy vegetables, fortified soy milk, and almonds are examples of some vegan calcium sources. The following table lists amounts of vegan foods that provide approximately 150 milligrams of calcium. By choosing at least six servings (6 × 150 = 900 milligrams) from this list and getting the rest of the calcium you need from other foods, you can meet the RDA of 1,000 milligrams of calcium. If you are taking a supplement that contains calcium, you will need fewer servings of calcium-rich foods.

Foods Supplying Approximately 150 Milligrams of Calcium

Food	Serving Size
Cooked collards or turnip greens	¾ cup
Cooked kale or broccoli rabe	1 cup
Cooked bok choy, okra, or mustard greens	1 cup
Cooked broccoli	2½ cups
Calcium-fortified juice (orange or vegetable) or milk (soy, almond, etc.)	4 ounces
Calcium-fortified vegan yogurt	3 ounces
Calcium-fortified vegan cheese	¾ ounce
Tofu	2 ounces
Tempeh	¾ cup
Almonds	6 tablespoons
Almond butter or tahini	2½ tablespoons
Cooked dried beans	1½ cups (1 cup soybeans)
Dried figs	10
English muffin made with calcium propionate	1½
Blackstrap molasses	2 teaspoons
Calcium-fortified energy bar	½

Meeting the Needs of Multiples

If you're carrying twins, triplets, or other multiples, you'll need more servings from all the food groups; your needs for calories and protein are higher. Protein needs for mothers of twins can be met by adding at least three servings of grains, two servings of protein-rich foods, and one serving of vegetables to the Vegan Food Guide for Pregnancy.

Menu Planning

Many women choose to eat three meals and several snacks during pregnancy to stave off hunger pangs and to keep from feeling uncomfortably full as the baby gets bigger. Remember, snacks don't have to be a big production. A piece of fruit and some nuts or trail mix can be a satisfying snack.

Here's a sample menu based on the Vegan Food Guide for Pregnancy:

BREAKFAST

- ½ cup oatmeal (1 serving grains)
- 2 tablespoons almond butter (1 serving protein; calcium source)
- 4 ounces calcium-fortified orange juice (1 serving fruit; calcium source)

MIDMORNING SNACK

- ½ bagel (1 serving grains)
- ½ cup hummus (1 serving protein; calcium source)

LUNCH

- Sandwich with 1 slice whole-wheat bread (1 serving grains), 1 ounce vegan deli slices (1 serving protein), and 1 teaspoon vegan mayonnaise (1 serving fats)
- 1 cup mixed greens (1 serving vegetables)
- Medium apple (1 serving fruit)

MIDAFTERNOON SNACK

- ¼ cup cashews (1 serving protein)
- 1 cup baby carrots (1 serving vegetables)

DINNER

- 1 cup pasta with tomato sauce (2 servings grains)
- ½ cup chickpeas (1 serving protein)
- 1 cup collards (2 servings vegetables; calcium source) with 1 teaspoon olive oil (1 serving fats)

BEDTIME SNACK

- 1 ounce ready-to-eat cereal (1 serving grains)
- 8 ounces calcium-fortified soy milk (2 servings protein; calcium source)

You'll probably need to add some more foods in order to support weight gain. This sample menu shows how to meet the minimum number of servings for the Vegan Food Guide for Pregnancy. Be sure to choose a variety of foods and use a daily prenatal supplement.

The Best Foods

Eating a variety of foods is always good advice. That way, if one food that you eat is high in vitamin X but low in mineral Y, you're likely to choose another food that will be low in vitamin X but high in mineral Y. Eating a variety of foods lets you relax and not have to worry about keeping track of every nutrient.

Certain foods in each food group are especially good sources of a variety of nutrients. For example, in the grains group, whole grains supply more fiber and more of some vitamins and minerals than their refined counterparts. In the vegetables group, dark-green vegetables and deep-orange vegetables are your best choice. That doesn't mean iceberg lettuce and mushrooms are off limits; it just means that these less nutrient-rich foods should be balanced with some kale and carrots.

Fresh fruits provide more fiber than more processed fruits or juices. If you choose to use canned fruits, select fruits packed in fruit juice rather than in heavy syrup. Dried beans, tofu, tempeh, soy milk, nuts, and nut butters are excellent choices from the protein-rich foods group. More processed foods like veggie "meats" are often higher in sodium, lower in fiber, and more expensive.

Foods to Limit

"Everything in moderation." It's a standard piece of nutrition advice that is important for vegans as well. While moderation is a reasonable approach to eating, be sure that you know what "moderation" means. It means that after you have eaten the appropriate amounts of nutrient-rich foods, it's all right to have a small (emphasis on small) amount of "junk foods."

You would be just fine, nutritionally speaking, if you never ate junk foods again. The sole nutritional value of these foods is that they provide calories; they're not great sources of protein, vitamins, minerals, or other things you need.

Examples of junk foods are soft drinks, candy, cookies, cake, chips, and greasy snack foods. Remember, just because a food is vegan doesn't mean it's healthy. What's wrong with these foods?

Think of your eating plan like your household budget—you have to make choices to stay on your budget. If you need a certain amount of calories to support weight gain in pregnancy, you don't want to "spend" those calories on non-nutritious foods. Rather, you want to get the best nutrition possible within your allotted calories. If you overdo junk foods, they can displace healthier foods in your diet—not good for you or your baby.

That said, if gaining enough weight is a struggle, judicious use of junk foods can help. Once you've eaten your day's share of healthy foods, you can add calories with some higher-calorie, lower-nutrient foods.

Finding the Time to Eat Right

Whether you're working a hectic job or home with young children or both, eating right can be a matter of planning ahead. If you're crunched for time, it may seem simpler to just skip a meal or grab something (anything) on the way out the door. Of course, there will be times when that's your only choice. Overall, however, setting up a plan can help you eat well.

Quick and Easy Meals

Having a collection of quick and easy meals in your repertoire can help when your plans to get home early and cook dinner don't pan out. Think of meals that you can make without a cookbook or special ingredients. Keep a stock of different breads and rolls in the freezer. A quick meal that has good nutrients is some hummus or other spread in a wrap with vegetables and a piece of fruit. Scrambled tofu is a quick meal to put together, especially if you have frozen or fresh vegetables that you can scramble along with the tofu. Look for quick-cooking pasta and keep either jarred or homemade sauce on hand. Keep a stock of veggie burgers and buns in the freezer. With canned vegetarian baked beans and some baby carrots, this is a superquick meal.

Some families use part of a weekend day to make several meals for the week or to do the prep for meals—chop vegetables, cook potatoes for potato salad later, bake bread or desserts. Make-ahead dishes like casseroles, soups, and stews can be refrigerated and then reheated on nights when there's not a lot of time to cook. Leftovers can be frozen and used in a few weeks to add variety. Be sure to keep a list of what's in your freezer so that you don't find mysterious ice-encrusted packages months later and wonder what they are.

Convenience Foods That Work for You

Foods labeled as "convenience foods" may make you think of junk foods that you dash into a convenience food store to buy and then eat as you drive. Actually, convenience foods are any foods that can make it easier for you to get a meal together quickly. Choosing good convenience foods and keeping them on hand is one way to ensure that your nutritional needs are met. Canned beans are an example of a useful convenience food that comes in many varieties. Give them a quick rinse to remove some of the canning brine's salt and then use them in any dish calling for cooked beans.

Precut or frozen vegetables can make it easier to serve vegetables. Look for bags of shredded cabbage or peeled winter squash if time is tight. Keeping frozen fruit on hand means it's easy to make smoothies or fruit crisps and to add fruit to muffins or pancakes.

Smart Snacking

Snacking is a key to getting the foods you need. When you are early in your pregnancy, snacks can help with your fickle appetite and with the need to keep nausea at bay by having food in your stomach. As your pregnancy progresses, you'll be less likely to have room for three large meals a day. Instead, you may choose to eat six or more small meals (aka snacks) daily.

Some snack ideas include:

- Fresh fruit or a fruit smoothie
- Vegetables with a tofu or bean dip
- Rice cakes or bagel slices with nut butter
- Cereal and soy milk
- Bran or blueberry muffin
- Trail mix
- Energy bar and fruit juice

All of these snack ideas involve minimal preparation time. Dips and muffins can be purchased or prepared on a day when you have time, then kept refrigerated or frozen to use as needed.

Vegan in a Nonvegan Family

Suppose that you are vegan but the rest of your household is not. You could microwave a veggie burger every night, but that's really not a solution. Your partner may want to try some vegan foods or even make some vegan meals for you. You need ideas for vegan foods that everyone will eat.

One approach that many vegans in this situation take is to make meatless dishes that you eat as entrées and that your partner can use as side dishes. Another idea is to make dishes you can eat as is and that your partner can add meat or cheese to. For example, stir-fried vegetables can be supplemented with sautéed tofu or chicken. Cheese or cooked ground beef can be added to pasta sauce or chili.

If you make burritos or tacos, your portion can be filled with beans and veggies and your partner's with meat or cheese. Similarly, baked potatoes can be topped with a bean-based or meat-based sauce.

Chapter 9

Vegan Shopping and Ingredients

Soy milk in the dairy case, tofu in the produce cooler, nondairy frozen desserts next to the ice cream—these days many supermarkets are carrying vegan foods. Depending on your location and your food preferences, you may be able to do all of your food shopping in your neighborhood store. Vegans also choose to shop at food co-ops and natural foods stores that may carry a greater variety of vegan specialty products. And if you'd prefer to grocery shop from home, there are a number of online vegan stores.

Finding Vegan Foods in a Supermarket

Your local supermarket carries an impressive number of vegan-friendly foods. While it may take some time to read labels at first, you'll quickly learn which foods and brands will work for you. You may find that most of your purchases are coming from several sections of the store—produce, canned and dried beans, and natural foods, perhaps. All of these sections will be places you'll find vegan foods, but if you're willing to explore, you'll find that most areas of the store have some vegan items.

Produce Section

It seems obvious that you'd be a regular in the fresh fruit and vegetable aisle. Besides being the place to find produce, the produce section is where many stores locate vegan and vegetarian items. Look around and you may find tofu, mock meats, dairy alternatives, and vegan salad dressings nearby. Be daring—challenge yourself to try a new fruit or vegetable every week or two. And get to know the produce manager; she can often help you decide if a fruit is ripe or provide ideas for using celeriac and other less common vegetables or fruits.

Deli Section

In many stores, the deli section is where you can find a variety of kinds of hummus as well as olives and pickles. Most brands of hummus are vegan, although it never hurts to check the ingredients list. Some stores have packages of vegan deli "meats" in this section. Prepared salads like coleslaw or potato salad are often made with egg-based mayonnaise, but don't be afraid to ask about vegan items—you may find a roasted potato salad with a vinaigrette dressing or a vegan shredded-vegetable salad. Besides, by asking, you are making the store employees aware that people are looking for vegan options.

Bakery Section

Finding vegan bread in a supermarket can be challenging. Many breads contain whey (milk derivative), eggs, or honey. Rye breads are usually vegan, as are some traditional French and Italian breads. You may have better luck at a store with a natural foods or ethnic section.

Grocery Section

The grocery section is one part of the store where you can find items you never realized were vegan. It's worthwhile to occasionally spend an hour or so in this section, reading labels and making notes of unexpected "finds." Here are some tips for approaching this section of the store:

- If you're looking for a cracker, steer clear of those with cheese or butter in the product's name. Crackers with whole-wheat flour as the first ingredient are a better choice than those with wheat flour listed first.
- Many canned fruits, beans, and vegetables are vegan. Check vegetable labels for added salt pork, bacon, or other meat ingredients. These are especially common in canned greens and beans.
- Hot cereals like oatmeal, grits, and polenta are often vegan. Often the plain (or original) version will simply have the grain as its ingredient. Check the labels on hot cereals for milk or cheese.
- Many brands of pasta are vegan. Some will have eggs added, especially noodles or fettuccine, so check the label. Pasta sauces may have meat or cheese added; marinara sauces are often vegan.
- The ethnic section of the grocery store can have some interesting items. Look for falafel mix in the Middle Eastern section, lard-free refried beans in the Hispanic section, and unusual dried noodles in the Asian section.
- Some supermarkets also have a natural foods section. Of course, all items are not vegan, but this may be where you will find aseptically packaged soy milk, vegan canned soups, and vegan breakfast cereals.
- While not the healthiest part of the store, the snacks aisle does include vegan potato chips, pretzels, tortilla chips, and other munchies. Watch for added cheese or other dairy products.

Frozen Foods Section

The frozen foods section is where you'll find frozen vegetables (great for times when the produce drawer is empty and your dinner needs a vegetable), frozen fruits (think smoothies), frozen juice concentrate, and, frequently, frozen veggie burgers. There may be other surprises like vegan pierogi, vegan soups, and vegan frozen desserts.

Dairy Section

Although you might not expect the dairy aisle to have vegan selections, this is where many supermarkets stock refrigerated soy milk and other plant milks. You may also find fruit juices in this section. In some well-stocked supermarkets, you'll also find nondairy yogurt and margarine.

Are frozen vegetables more nutritious than fresh? It depends. Frozen vegetables are frequently processed immediately after they're picked to minimize nutrient loss. After harvesting, vegetables lose vitamins with exposure to air and sunlight. So if the fresh broccoli is several days away from when it was picked, it may be significantly lower in some vitamins than frozen broccoli.

If you have favorite vegan products that you've seen in other stores or heard about in magazines or online, ask the manager of your supermarket if it would be possible to stock these. If it's a product you know you like and will use, the manager may be able to order a case for you.

Label Reading

What if you could quickly glance at a food's label and know immediately whether or not it is vegan? Such a simple scheme doesn't really exist today, at least not in any consistent way. The US government does not regulate or require the word *vegan* on food labels. If you see a product labeled "vegan" or some sort of an identification mark, it's probably because either the food company or a nonprofit organization has decided that this product meets its standards. It's more likely you'll need to take a look at the ingredient listing to see if a product meets your criteria to be included in your grocery cart.

Some obvious signs that a food isn't vegan is that it contains meat, fish, poultry, egg, or dairy ingredients. Then there are ingredients like gelatin, beef broth, lard, and Worcestershire sauce (contains anchovies) that are derived from meat or fish. Dairy-derived ingredients include casein (milk protein), whey, and lactase (milk sugar). Some ingredients sound like they might be dairy derived but aren't, like cocoa butter, cream of tartar, and lactic acid.

> If an ingredient listing contains the term *natural flavors,* the United States Department of Agriculture (USDA) Food Safety and Inspection Service requires that the label indicate if the natural flavors are derived from animal sources. The term *natural flavors* on a label without additional qualification means spices, spice extracts, or essential oils were used to flavor the food.

If you have questions about an ingredient and whether or not it is vegan, contact the food company. The company may not be able to tell you, but if it receives the question enough, it'll start checking with its ingredient suppliers and may even try to use nonanimal ingredients.

Natural Foods Stores, Food Co-Ops, the Internet, and More

If you have a natural foods store or a food co-op nearby, chances are good that you'll find many vegan products on the shelves and in the bulk food bins. Look for all different kinds of dried beans and grains as well as a variety of vegan mock meats and dairy alternatives. Of course, not all foods in these stores are vegan, so label reading is in order. Some seemingly natural products are derived from animals or insects. Did you know that the red color of some juices and candies comes from the dried bodies of female insects? If you'd like to avoid this, don't buy products with carmine or cochineal as an ingredient.

Natural foods stores and food co-ops often have bulk food bins. These are a great way to try a small amount of a new food or spice. If you have allergies, however, beware—cross contamination from one bulk bin to another is highly likely.

> The FDA requires that food labels clearly identify all ingredients derived from the most common food allergens: milk, eggs, fish, shellfish, tree nuts, peanuts, wheat, and soybeans. A product that does not list any of these is not necessarily vegan since it could contain meat.

Just like supermarkets, natural foods stores and food co-ops are often happy to order items for you. If you don't see what you want, talk to a manager.

Vegans living in areas with limited shopping options as well as vegans who like to support vegan-owned companies often look to web-based businesses. Several companies sell only products that they identify as vegan—everything from vegan chocolate to vegan skin-care products and cosmetics. Even refrigerated and frozen items can be shipped.

Prices for products ordered online are often similar to those in stores, but you do have the addition of shipping costs. To save, look for special promotions or combine your order with a friend's to get a volume discount. Appendix A includes examples of some online shopping resources.

Stores catering to ethnic populations can yield exciting foods for vegans. Asian grocery stores often carry mock meats, sauces, noodles, rice, exotic vegetables, and other delights. Kosher food stores often carry dairy substitutes. Stores carrying Indian products may have more varieties of dried beans and rice than you have ever seen, along with fragrant spices.

People who follow the Seventh-day Adventist religion are encouraged to eat a vegetarian diet. Adventists, as they are called, have a long history of developing creative vegetarian foods, especially mock meats. Adventist stores carry several brands of canned and frozen products, many of which are vegan. If you're wishing for vegan scallops, ham, or chops, you will probably find these soy- or wheat-based products in an Adventist store.

Wherever you live, you can find a generous supply of vegan foods. Although specialty stores can add variety, even in small-town USA you can buy the grains, beans, fruits, and vegetables that are vegan staples.

Shopping on a Budget

Being vegan can result in a drop in your weekly grocery bill, especially if you're choosing beans and whole grains to replace steaks and lobster. However, if you are buying a lot of vegan specialty or convenience foods, you may see an increase in your food costs. But it doesn't have to cost more to be a vegan.

Plan Ahead

While convenience foods and takeout can be lifesavers on nights you just can't face the stove, a steady diet of these foods can drive up food costs. Planning ahead doesn't necessarily mean having detailed menus for every meal (although you can do this), but it does mean having some quickly prepared foods in your cupboard or refrigerator. Inexpensive foods to keep on hand for quick meals include tofu, canned beans, and pasta. Taking a few minutes before your regular grocery store trip to check that you have staple foods on the shelf or on your list can save you from multiple trips to the store—costly in terms of time and money if you tend to impulse shop.

Cook It Yourself

Planning ahead also makes it more likely you'll be able to cook more of your own food. That way you can save for a splurge night out at a favorite restaurant rather than eating less-than-tasty takeout just because it's convenient. Maybe it makes sense to do most of your cooking on days when you and your partner are home. Perhaps you can make several dinners and put them in the freezer or refrigerator for later in the week.

Cooking a large pot of beans and one of grains on the weekend can give you the basics for several meals—stir-fry some vegetables one night, toss in some beans, and serve over the grain; another night, combine beans, grains, and a vegan salad dressing for a quick entrée salad. If you like to experiment, try making your own seitan or baking your own bread. Along with cost savings, you'll also have learned a new skill.

Shop Smart

Many vegan staples aren't that expensive. Foods like dried beans and grains are relatively low cost. Specialty foods, including plant milks, mock meats, nut butters, and frozen convenience foods, can take a chunk out of your food budget. If these foods are important to you, there are some ways to cut costs. Store brands of some specialty foods are available, cost less, and are often of comparable quality compared to name brands. For example, many stores sell their own brand of soy milk at a significantly lower price. Many stores, especially smaller stores or food co-ops, offer a case discount of 10 percent or so. If it's a food you'll be able to use before the expiration date, talk to the manager about purchasing a case or more. When products you use are on sale, stock up. If you have space to store them, you can get six months' worth of your favorite brand of chickpeas or vegan canned soup when it's on sale.

Vegan Ingredients

While specialty items are not an essential part of a vegan diet, some of these foods can add variety or even serve as an easy source of some nutrients. Tofu and soy milk may once have seemed exotic, but now they're showing up in many mainstream supermarkets. Other less familiar foods that you may see in recipes and wonder about include seitan, agave, and flaxseeds.

Soy Products

All soy products are made from soybeans. Soybeans are a high-protein bean native to East Asia. They are sold in fresh, frozen, canned, and dried forms. Edamame are a special soybean variety and are sweeter than traditional soybeans. They look a bit like lima beans and are found in the frozen foods section. Fresh edamame are sometimes found at farmers' markets and in the produce section. Soybeans should not be eaten raw; cooking makes them more digestible.

Soy milk is made by soaking, grinding, and straining soybeans. It is available in both shelf-stable and refrigerated forms and comes in flavors like vanilla, chocolate, and carob. In mid-December, you can sometimes find eggnog-flavored soy milk. Vegans often rely on fortified soy milk as a source of calcium, vitamin B_{12}, and vitamin D, so check the label of the brand you prefer to make sure these important nutrients have been added.

Unflavored soy milk is mixed with a coagulant to make tofu in a process that is similar to making cheese. For best results, choose the right kind of tofu for the dish you'll be using it in. Silken tofu (often available in shelf-stable packaging) is best used for dishes where you want a creamy consistency—shakes, puddings, salad dressings, and pie fillings. Firm or extra-firm tofu is a better choice for stir-fries and other dishes where you want the tofu to keep its shape. Once a package of refrigerated tofu is opened, any unused tofu should be refrigerated and covered with water. Change the water at least every other day. Discard opened, unused tofu after 5 to 7 days or when it exceeds the expiration date on the package, whichever comes first. Shelf-stable tofu should be refrigerated after opening for no more than 5 to 7 days but not to exceed the expiration date. Shelf-stable tofu does not need to be covered with water.

Tempeh, a popular addition to soups and casseroles, originated in Indonesia. Tempeh is made from whole soybeans that have been fermented, either alone or with a grain. Tempeh has a crumbly texture that some find reminds them of meat.

TVP is made from soy flour. It is often found in the bulk section of natural foods stores. TVP is sold in chunks and granules and may be flavored to taste like beef or chicken. TVP must be soaked in boiling water to rehydrate it. It can then be used in chilis, sloppy joes, spaghetti sauces, and other recipes in place of ground beef.

Wheat Meat and Other "Not Meats"

If you've eaten in a vegetarian Chinese restaurant, you've probably eaten seitan. Seitan is made from gluten, the protein part of wheat. It has a chewy texture and can be baked, boiled, or stir-fried. Seitan, also called *wheat meat*, can be found in the refrigerated section of natural foods stores. You can also make your own seitan; a gluten flour mix makes it easy.

These days you can find a vegan version of almost any meat or seafood product. These "not meats" are often made from soy or seitan, although other beans and grains are sometimes used, especially in veggie burgers. Check labels—some have eggs, egg whites, or cheese added.

From Thanksgiving "unturkey" to Fourth of July veggie dogs, there are products for every occasion. These products are often high in protein and may be fortified with iron, zinc, or vitamin B_{12}. The downside is that they tend to be expensive.

Nut and Seed Butters

Nut and seed butters add protein, calories, and essential fats to vegan diets. Well-stocked stores feature almond butter, hazelnut butter, cashew butter, macadamia butter, and more. They can be used for sandwiches; to add richness to a smoothie; or to flavor soups, stews, and grain dishes. For those with nut allergies, try soy nut butter (made from roasted soybeans), sunflower seed butter, and tahini (sesame seed butter). Even if you still prefer peanut butter, check out some of the flavored peanut butters—from spicy to cinnamon-raisin.

Move Over, Milk

Besides the previously mentioned soy milk, many other plant milks are available based on hemp seeds, almonds, oats, rice, coconut, and more. Which one you choose is a personal preference, although if you are relying on plant milks as sources of key nutrients, be aware that not all are fortified and check the labels to find one that meets your needs. Soy milk is highest in protein with 6–10 grams of protein in a cup. Oat milk and hemp milk have about half as much protein, and rice, coconut, and almond milks provide only about 1 gram of protein per cup. Unflavored, original, or plain varieties of plant milks work best in savory dishes. Flavored milks (vanilla, chocolate, carob, and others) are sweeter and work in desserts and drinks.

Vegan cheese is typically made from rice, soybeans, peas, or nuts. It can be used in recipes that call for dairy cheese, but it does not have the same nutritional profile. Some brands of vegan cheese do have calcium added. Most are quite low in protein. Grating or shredding vegan cheese helps it melt and combine with other ingredients.

Vegan yogurt can be found in the dairy case of supermarkets and natural foods stores. Yogurt is commonly made from soy milk; coconut milk–based yogurt is a recent addition. Several brands of vegan yogurt are fortified with vitamins and minerals to resemble dairy yogurt.

> Packages of nondairy cheese that say "lactose-free" but do not say "vegan" or "casein-free" frequently contain casein, a protein that comes from cow's milk. Casein is what gives cheese its stretchy quality when melted. Cheese that contains casein is not vegan. Some brands of vegan cheese use other ingredients to mimic casein's stretchiness.

No Yolk (or White Either)

Commercial egg replacers containing various binding agents are often used to replace eggs in vegan baking. Ground flaxseeds can be blended with water and used as egg replacers. A tablespoon and a half of ground flaxseeds blended with ¼ cup of water can substitute for a large egg. You can purchase whole flaxseeds and grind them yourself or purchase them already ground (flaxseed meal). Opened packages of flaxseed should be stored in the refrigerator or freezer.

For Your Sweet Tooth

Vegans with a sweet tooth can find all sorts of vegan chocolates, baked goods, and frozen desserts at vegan bakeries and candy stores, natural foods stores, and online. It's also easy to make your own desserts.

A Few Other Ingredients

Nutritional yeast is used in vegan recipes to add a cheese flavor. It can be sprinkled on popcorn or vegetables. This is not brewer's yeast, which has a bitter flavor. You'll know it's nutritional yeast if you see pale-yellow flakes or granules. Red Star Vegetarian Support Formula (VSF) Yeast Flakes nutritional yeast is a reliable source of vitamin B_{12}.

If you're buying nutritional yeast from the bulk food bin and relying on that to supply your vitamin B_{12}, check often to make sure the store is selling the vitamin

B_{12}–rich form—you can definitely buy nutritional yeast that does not supply vitamin B_{12}.

If you have a favorite recipe that calls for honey or you like something sweet to add to herbal tea, you might try agave nectar. Agave nectar is a liquid sweetener produced from the juice of a succulent plant. Agave nectar mainly provides sugar and calories, so it should be used in moderation.

Eating Organically Produced Foods

Many vegans choose to purchase at least some organically produced foods. If you're pregnant, you may be even more likely to seek out these foods, hoping it will help give your baby a healthy start. Just what is it that makes a food organic?

Organic foods are grown without using most conventional pesticides and fertilizers. A product that is identified as being organic is not produced by genetic engineering. Ionizing radiation and sewage sludge cannot be used in organic production or handling. Organic farming practices include soil and water conservation measures. Crop rotation, manure, and compost are used to improve the soil in place of using conventional fertilizers. Instead of using commercial insecticides or herbicides, organic farmers might use companion planting to discourage insects, and they might use mulch and hand weeding to control weeds.

Researchers continue to debate whether or not organically produced foods are more nutritious than conventionally grown products. Organic practices do benefit the environment as well as farm workers who are not exposed to potentially harmful pesticides and herbicides. Some people say that organic food tastes better.

The food label will tell you whether a product is organic or not. The USDA is responsible for the organic labeling program and allows one of three possible labels:

- Products labeled "100 percent organic" must contain only organically produced ingredients.
- Products labeled "organic" must have at least 95 percent of their ingredients organically produced.
- Products labeled "made with organic ingredients" must contain at least 70 percent organic ingredients.

Products that contain less than 70 percent organic ingredients can list individual ingredients as organic but cannot say that the product is organic.

Organic produce can be costlier than conventional produce. To reduce costs, buy locally and in season. If you can afford to purchase only some organic foods, focus on those where you don't remove the outer skin. Products where the thick peel or rind is removed before eating probably contain lower levels of pesticides than foods where the entire product, skin and all, is eaten. Think lemons versus apples, for example.

Eating Locally Grown Foods

Locally grown food has the advantage of being freshly picked. It has not been on a truck or in a warehouse for days before getting to the store. The farmer may have to drive his beets only five miles to the market rather than having them fly for thousands of miles from another country.

Another way to support your local farmer is to join a Community Supported Agriculture (CSA) farm. In the CSA model, a farmer sells shares in her farm. You (the shareholder) receive a weekly supply of fruits and vegetables from the farm. You may go to a central location to pick up your share, or it may be delivered to your house. Your CSA may include picking privileges—in season you can pick your own strawberries, green beans, cherry tomatoes, herbs, and more. Many CSAs feature organic produce. Although a CSA requires a considerable outlay ahead of the farming season, you then get many months of produce at no additional cost.

Once the baby comes, or if you have children already, trips to farms or farmers' markets are fun family outings that let your children see where their food comes from.

Chapter 10

Eating and Drinking Safely

You know what you need to eat, but did you know that there are some foods that should be avoided during pregnancy? Some of these foods (or beverages) contain substances that could be potentially harmful. Others have a higher likelihood of being contaminated with microorganisms that can cause foodborne illness. You may need to change some of your shopping habits and food prep techniques to reduce the risk of foodborne illness. Learning some of these safe food-handling habits now will help later when you're preparing baby or toddler meals.

Foodborne Illness

Every year the CDC estimates about one out of six Americans develops foodborne illness. Foodborne illness, also called food poisoning, is caused by eating food or drinking beverages that are contaminated with microorganisms—bacteria, viruses, or parasites. A foodborne illness can cause vomiting, diarrhea, and stomach cramps. Other symptoms are flu-like—fever, muscle aches, and headache.

Besides being an unpleasant experience, a foodborne illness is an especially important concern in pregnancy. First of all, simply being pregnant increases your risk of developing a foodborne illness. Your immune system is not as active during pregnancy, so you're not as able to hold off bacteria and other contaminants. Your unborn baby's immune system is not mature enough to protect him from microorganisms.

Symptoms of foodborne illness can occur as soon as about twenty minutes after eating the contaminated food to as long as six weeks later. Most foodborne illnesses appear in one to three days, however, and last a few days. Some can leave you feeling ill for a longer time.

A second concern with a foodborne illness is that it can cause serious problems, including miscarriage or premature delivery. Sometimes, even when your symptoms are mild, your baby can be negatively affected. Fortunately, there are some very specific steps you can take to reduce your risk of foodborne illness.

If, despite your best efforts, you think you have a foodborne illness, contact your healthcare provider immediately. Your blood may need to be tested to see what is causing your illness. You may need help staying hydrated if you have vomiting or diarrhea. Your doctor may prescribe an antibiotic that is safe to use in pregnancy. If you think your illness was from food you ate away from home, also contact the health department in your community so it can investigate the restaurant to reduce the risk of other people getting sick.

Foods to Avoid

Some foods should be completely off the menu in pregnancy because of their higher risk of contamination with microorganisms that could make you ill. Many of the foods on standard lists of foods to avoid are not vegan—raw eggs, undercooked meat, raw milk, soft cheeses, sushi, and some fish, for example. Vegans do have to be aware of some potential food-safety issues, however. Foods that should be avoided in pregnancy include raw sprouts of any kind and unpasteurized juice or cider. Raw sprouts are on the list of foods to avoid because potentially harmful bacteria can get into the sprout seeds before they are sprouted. Once bacteria are inside the seed's shell, it is very difficult to eliminate them. If you are eating out, ask that raw sprouts not be added to your sandwich or salad.

Fresh-squeezed juice, purchased in the supermarket or at a juice bar, may not be pasteurized. Pasteurization involves heating the juice to a temperature hot enough to reduce the number of microorganisms. Unpasteurized juices or cider should be avoided when you are pregnant.

The good news if you're vegan is that you don't have to worry about raw eggs in vegan cookie dough or raw fish in vegan sushi. Lunch meats often show up on the "to be avoided" lists, but vegan lunch meats are all right to eat.

If your kitchen is used to prepare meat, you'll need to take some precautions to make sure your food is not contaminated with microorganisms from the meat.

Kitchen Safety

Proper storage and handling of food, from the supermarket to your dinner table, is the best way to combat foodborne illness in your kitchen. On shopping day, make sure you check expiration labels before you buy. And because changes in storage temperature can breed bacteria in many foods, shop for refrigerated and frozen foods last and make sure they're the first items to be put away when you get home.

Safe Food Preparation

Your mom always told you to wash your hands before you started preparing foods, and she was right. Hands need to be washed with soap and warm water before and after handling food, and after using the bathroom, changing a diaper, or handling a pet.

Food Safety If You Live with a Nonvegan

Even if you are a staunch vegan, you may be living with others who eat meat, fish, or poultry. Whether they prepare their own food or you make a meat meal for them and a vegan meal for yourself, it's important that everyone is clear on proper food handling.

Interested in canning fruits and vegetables from your garden, CSA, or farmers' market? Make sure you preserve food safely. Visit the National Center for Home Food Preservation at https://nchfp.uga.edu for research-based information about methods of home food preservation. This website also offers the USDA's *Complete Guide to Home Canning*, fact sheets, and consumer bulletins.

If you share a kitchen with someone who eats meat, be sure that all raw meat, poultry, and seafood are double-wrapped and stored in a separate area of the refrigerator to prevent any juices from contaminating other foods. These raw foods should also be isolated from other foods during meal preparation. Keep your refrigerator clean and wipe up spills immediately when they occur to discourage bacteria growth.

When someone in your household prepares raw meat, eggs, poultry, fish, or shellfish, all knives, dishes, cutting boards, food prep surfaces, and utensils that come in contact with the food need to be immediately and thoroughly cleaned. Try not to use the same cutting board for raw meat and fruits and vegetables. Hands should be washed with hot, soapy water. A clean set of utensils and serving dishes needs to be used with the cooked food.

Fruit and Vegetable Safety

Fruits and vegetables should also get a good cleaning. Thoroughly rinse everything you get from the produce stand and your own garden. Even veggies that are precut and packaged should be washed again before eating. If you're doing your own vegetable or fruit gardening, do not use untreated manure, as it may harbor pathogens that could contaminate your fruits and vegetables.

Tofu Safety

Tofu is a perishable food, so make sure that the store where you purchase it keeps the tofu refrigerated and not tucked in with the vegetable display. Some markets or food co-ops may still sell bulk tofu in buckets of water—you select your tofu and place it in a container for purchase. There are many opportunities for this tofu to be contaminated, so avoid this kind of tofu when you are pregnant. Individually packaged tofu is a safer option; just be sure to use it before the expiration date. If you use only part of a package, place the remaining tofu in a clean container, cover with water (unless it is a shelf-stable version), and refrigerate and use within five to seven days, not to exceed the expiration date. Change the water at least every other day.

> Soy products, used in moderation, can make a significant nutrient contribution to a vegan diet.

Tofu that you plan to eat without cooking (for instance, tofu used to make a smoothie or a sandwich spread) should be steamed five to ten minutes before use. This extra step is usually not needed, but when you're pregnant, it's best to be safe.

Aseptically packaged tofu has been heat treated, so it does not need to be refrigerated before being opened. It also does not need to be steamed, even if you do plan to eat it without any additional cooking. Leftover aseptically packaged tofu should be refrigerated in a clean container and used within a few days.

Food Storage

When it's time to put away the leftovers, make sure you seal them up tightly and immediately refrigerate them. Leftovers should only be reheated once, to a temperature of 165°F (use a kitchen thermometer to check the temperature in the middle of the food).

Other Food Safety Issues

The bread that you bought a few days ago has blue fuzzy spots, the peaches you picked up for a pie are soft and have a white film, and the potatoes in the vegetable drawer have a greenish tinge. What's safe and what should be discarded? Some molds can make you sick if you eat them. Some can cause breathing problems or allergic reactions. Not uncommonly, moldy food is also contaminated with bacteria.

Using foods shortly after purchase, checking for expiration dates, and keeping refrigerated foods covered are all ways to prevent mold growth. If you do discover moldy food, however, avoid smelling it to keep from inhaling the mold. Discard any food that is covered with mold and check any nearby items that the moldy food has touched. One moldy carrot can spread mold to other foods in the vegetable drawer.

Although it may seem simple to just cut out the moldy part of a food, this may not eliminate all parts of the mold. Molds send out "roots" that go below the food's surface. Getting rid of the mold can be difficult. It's best to just toss what has gone moldy for safety's sake.

Small mold spots on firm fruits and vegetables with low moisture content (cabbage, broccoli stem, carrots) can be carefully cut off. Keep the knife out of the mold and cut off at least 1" around the mold spot. Soft fruits and vegetables with a high moisture content (peaches, tomatoes, cucumbers, strawberries) that are moldy should be discarded. Any other foods with mold, including jelly, bread, leftovers, and veggie "meats," should be safely discarded.

Greenish potatoes can be contaminated with a toxic substance called *solanine*. Solanine can be fatal at high levels and can cause nausea, vomiting, and diarrhea. To be safe, discard potatoes with a greenish color or that taste bitter.

Dining Out

You can't ensure safe handling and preparation of your meals when you're not in control of the kitchen. But treating yourself to the occasional night out at a restaurant is perhaps even more important now that you're pregnant. When possible, go to restaurants you know and trust. When dining somewhere new, stick with safe menu choices that are less likely to harbor foodborne illness, such as pasta. Avoid anything sold off a cart or truck, and steer clear of eateries that look poorly kept and dirty (chances are the kitchens are too).

When your meal is done, skip the doggie bag. Food should be refrigerated within two hours—counting from the moment the cook sticks it under the heat lamp. Allowing for a leisurely meal, a reasonably efficient waitstaff, and travel time home from the restaurant, it's more than likely you won't make the cutoff (unless you live above the restaurant or close to it)—giving your leftovers time to incubate bacteria.

Caffeine and Artificial Sweeteners

Caffeine sources range from coffee and tea to cocoa, chocolate, some soft drinks, energy drinks, and some over-the-counter medicines. While moderate caffeine intake of about 200 milligrams a day (about 12 ounces of coffee) does not seem to increase the risk of miscarriage or premature birth, studies are conflicting and researchers cannot say with certainty what a safe level of caffeine in pregnancy is. Caffeine can also increase the number of trips you make to the bathroom, according to the American Pregnancy Association.

You may be wondering about drinking diet sodas or using artificial sweeteners when you are pregnant. The FDA has determined that both aspartame (NutraSweet) and sucralose (Splenda) are safe for most people to use in moderation. The exceptions are anyone diagnosed with hyperphenylalaninemia (high levels of phenylalanine—a component of aspartame—in the bloodstream), with the genetic disease phenylketonuria (PKU), or with advanced liver disease.

Diet sodas can contain significant amounts of caffeine and can make you feel so full that you have little appetite for healthy foods. If you regularly drink diet sodas, consider cutting down or replacing them with water.

Chapter 11

Living Vegan While Pregnant

You may have a large circle of like-minded vegan friends or you may not know any other vegans. Regardless, you're probably aware that the majority of the world is not vegan. Social issues crop up—dinners with coworkers, holiday celebrations, visits to circuses and zoos. Being pregnant can complicate things as well. Will the baby be vegan? Can you be healthy and be vegan while you're pregnant? A few basic ideas will help you as you strive to be true to your vegan ideals.

Skeptical Friends

Your friends were used to your vegan diet when it was just you, but now you're going to be a mom. It seems like every time that you get together, your friends want to talk about your eating habits and whether or not you're eating enough protein or whatever else your baby needs. Sound familiar? Everyone seems to have a horror story about a friend of a friend who was vegan when she was pregnant and who ran into problems. How can you deal with all of this?

What's Really Going On?

Your friends care about you and want what's best for you. They need to know that you're thinking about good nutrition and getting what your baby requires. They want to be reassured that you have done your homework and that you know what you're doing. Your friends' eyes would probably start to glaze over if you walked them through every vitamin, mineral, and gram of protein you need and provided excruciating details about how you were going to do all of this. What's more important is that you calmly let them know that you're on top of things and that you're eating well, even if you are eating differently from them.

Options

If your friends are starting to get on your nerves with constant comments about your diet, you have several options. You may choose to use one or more of these possibilities, depending on the situation and how you otherwise feel about the friendship.

Although people may think that women are more often vegetarian, surveys—such as those conducted by The Vegetarian Resource Group in 2016—typically find that about half of adult vegetarians are men. According to The Vegetarian Resource Group, while vegetarians live everywhere, they're more likely to live in the western United States and the Northeast than in the Midwest.

Option One: Educate them. Remember, your friends are looking for reassurance that you're making good choices. Let them know that you've been reading about vegan pregnancy and that your healthcare provider is aware of your diet. You might mention positive things you're doing—taking a prenatal supplement, using fortified soy milk, cutting down on the junk food. Be ready to change the subject when necessary so that your eating habits do not become the sole topic of conversation.

Option Two: Agree to disagree. You've done your best to help your friend understand why you're eating the way you are and how you're making sure you're eating a healthy diet. In spite of everything, your friend continues to fret about your diet. A calm statement that lets your friend know that you appreciate her concern, you are convinced you're making good choices, and she's going to have to trust you on this one may be what's needed. Then change the subject.

Option Three: Let the friendship lapse. This may be the best choice if you find, despite your best efforts, that your eating habits are becoming the main focus of any encounter with a friend. Maybe this friendship will resume later; maybe it won't. In the meantime, be sure that you do have a support network of other friends.

Option Four: Seek out like-minded people. It may be time to look for some new friends. Maybe you'll find another vegan parent that you can commiserate with. Maybe you'll find a friend who's not vegan but has similar values to yours and who is comfortable with vegan diets.

Concerned Family Members

Just like your friends, your family may have gotten used to your vegan diet before you were pregnant. Now, however, they're expressing more concerns. They worry about protein and iron and whether you're eating enough. Actually, whether or not you're vegan, family members may seem to hover more when you're pregnant. If they weren't worrying about your diet, they might be worrying about how much work you're doing, or you continuing to exercise, or something else.

What's Really Going On?

Family members want what's best for you and for the baby. Just like friends, they want to know that you're making good choices. They may be concerned that you're not eating foods they think of as good foods for pregnancy—maybe foods that are traditional to their culture or that they ate when they were pregnant. They may worry that they won't be able to help you after the baby comes because they won't be able to make vegan food. They may be wondering if, a few years from now, they'll be able to make food for your child or children.

Making It Work

The third option for dealing with friends—letting the friendship lapse—is not really an option for family members. In order to figure out how to work with them, try to understand what they're really asking when they question your eating habits.

Some vegans have found that calmly providing supporting materials for their families to read is helpful. Perhaps show them a website from a reputable organization (see Appendix A). Find out what their concerns are and address them. Let them know that you've discussed your diet with your healthcare provider and with an RD, if you've done that.

Let your family know that you're not rejecting them; you just don't want to eat some of the foods that they eat. If they like to cook, this may be the time to share recipes with them or to invite them over so that you can show them how you make a simple dish or two. If your mom or mother-in-law collects cookbooks, give her a simple vegan cookbook—not because you expect her to become vegan but because you want her to be able to make vegan food if she wants to make food for you (and later for your child or children).

Nonvegan Partner

You're vegan; your partner isn't. Up until now, you've peacefully coexisted. Now, things are getting more confusing. How will the baby be raised? What will your child think if Mom eats one way and Dad another? There's no one-size-fits-all solution to these kinds of questions. As with other sensitive issues, your practices as a family will evolve and will be discussed over and over again.

More immediately, however, your partner may have the same concerns that friends and other family members have: Is it safe for you to be vegan? Will the baby's nutritional needs be met? Similar strategies to those you're using for friends and family apply to your partner as well. You can provide factual information and reassurance. You can encourage your partner to discuss concerns with your health-care provider. Maybe you really haven't been eating that well, and hearing your partner's concerns is the push you need to pay more attention. You can propose a consultation with an RD who can help you and your partner plan meals that will meet your needs.

Vegan Etiquette

Whether it's the restaurant that thinks fish is a vegan option or the friends who tell you that the soup has "just a little chicken broth in it," vegans are faced with some challenging social situations. You're often walking the line between advocating for your needs and realizing that other people are clueless about what those needs are.

Dining Out

Here's the scenario: Your coworkers want to take you out to lunch to celebrate your pregnancy. They know you are vegan, but you really haven't told them about what that means. They are suggesting going to an Italian restaurant, thinking it will have food you can eat. When you check with the restaurant ahead of time, you learn that the pasta is made with eggs, all sauces have cheese in them, and that you can have steamed broccoli and a plain salad. What should you do? You know a good vegan restaurant, but you're afraid it may seem too strange to your very mainstream coworkers.

You have several options. You can go with your colleagues to the restaurant and smile while you eat a plate of lettuce. Your coworkers will probably feel bad and wonder why you're not eating something more. They may be concerned that they've offended you. It may be better to suggest another restaurant—either the vegan restaurant if your coworkers are adventurous types or a compromise place that has vegan options for you and familiar dishes for your office mates. A Chinese restaurant may be a good compromise if you feel confident it will have vegan foods. Let your colleagues know how much you appreciate the offer to go out to lunch and that you don't expect them to know the ins and outs of your diet. Tell them that you checked with the restaurant they suggested, and it has very little that you can eat but that you know another restaurant you think would work. Enjoy your lunch!

Family Events

Scenario: Your mom has been making your birthday cakes your whole life. You've recently become vegan and don't want to hurt her feelings, but you don't want her usual death-by-chocolate cake made with six eggs and two sticks of butter. What to do?

First of all, let your mom know how much you love her and how much you treasure the memories of all the cakes she's made for you. Talk to her well in advance of your birthday so she has time to work with you on possible ideas. Help her understand how important being vegan is to you and how that affects the kind of birthday cake you have.

In place of cow's milk in vegan baking, you can use the same amount of plant-based milk. Milks can be soured to use in recipes calling for buttermilk by adding 1 tablespoon of lemon juice or vinegar to each cup of milk and letting it sit for a few minutes.

If your mom is open to it, suggest a good (and easy) vegan cake recipe that doesn't require a lot of exotic ingredients. See the dessert section of this book or vegan blogs or cookbooks for ideas. Don't be afraid to think outside the box. There's no rule that you have to celebrate a birthday with cake. If your mom is famous for another vegan dessert (maybe apple or peach pie), that might be a good choice for a birthday celebration. A store-bought cake is another idea. If you know a good vegan bakery, you could suggest that your family share a cake with you this year. This could be a good option if the idea of making a vegan cake is stressful for your mom.

Social Occasions

Here's the scenario: You've been invited to a baby shower for a friend. Your host has not mentioned any vegan food. In fact, you're not even sure the host knows you are vegan. Should you say something?

Put yourself in the host's position. Wouldn't you want to know if a guest had special needs? That's part of being a good host. As a good guest, you can make things easier for your host. Call ahead of time and explain your situation in very simple terms. Offer to bring a vegan dish to share. If the host tells you the menu, point out items that are vegan—maybe fruit salad or chips and salsa. If you're not sure there will be a lot of food you can eat and the host declines your offer to bring something, eat before you go and then fill a plate with food you can eat.

Holidays

Many family holidays revolve around food. And whether it's the Thanksgiving turkey, the Passover brisket, or the Fourth of July barbecue, the food is often not vegan.

Thanksgiving is a harvest festival, so think of dishes that feature seasonal foods. Ideas include a winter squash stuffed with wild rice and vegetables; roasted vegetables; stuffed peppers; a vegan quiche; tamale pie; or curried chickpeas and potatoes. You could also go with a homemade or purchased vegan "unturkey."

Your options include:

- Attend the family celebration and eat any vegan side dishes. Not a bad choice if you're comfortable with socializing with your family while they eat meat.
- Bring a vegan entrée to share. You'll still have to face the meat, but you'll have something more substantial to eat than side dishes. There's always the chance that other people will choose the vegan entrée over the meat entrée.

- Say you'll be able to come for dessert and bring a vegan dessert to share. You won't have to look at the meat, but you'll miss a part of your family gathering.
- Decide you'd prefer to have vegan holiday celebrations at your house and join your family for nonfood events or invite them to join you if they're okay with being vegan for the meal.

You have to decide which of these solutions, or others not listed, are most workable for your situation. Remember also that things change. Perhaps a relative's health issues will make your family more open to vegan celebrations in the future. Perhaps you'll feel less inclined to be at celebrations centered around meat when you have a young vegan. Do your best, and remember, it's not a vegan world.

Thinking Ahead

As you think ahead to having a child, you may be wondering how vegan families handle social events like birthday parties. Each family decides for itself how vegan their child or children will be. Some families send their child to parties with a vegan cupcake and a pint of vegan ice cream. Some families find that other parents are happy to make a vegan cake, especially if the circle of friends also includes children with dairy or egg allergies. Some families decide that it's all right for their child to eat vegetarian at birthday parties and stay vegan at home. What's right for your family may change over time as your child becomes more aware of why he is vegan and is able to express his desires. There will be many situations where you'll have to make choices for your child.

Finding Other Vegans

You realize that you'd like to get to know other vegans. Maybe it's because socializing would be easier if you didn't have to bring a vegan entrée to make sure you have something to eat. Maybe you'd like to learn more about how other people do things or swap ideas for food or pregnancy or children. Maybe you'd just like to expand your circle of friends. Social networking sites can help, as can old-fashioned word of mouth.

Local Vegan Groups

Many communities have groups of vegans or vegetarians that meet regularly. Groups may have potluck dinners, host speakers, go out to a restaurant together, or plan for animal-related activities. To find a group in your area, look for calendar listings in the local newspaper. Check bulletin boards at natural foods stores, vegetarian restaurants, and food co-ops. Contact area colleges or universities to see if there is a group on campus—they're often open to community members. National vegetarian organizations often have lists of local groups on their websites. You may see that a vegan cooking class is being offered at a store, restaurant, or school in your area. And, if there's not a local group, consider starting one.

National Vegan Groups

National vegan groups often hold conferences and exhibitions. If you live in or near a large city, you may be able to attend or volunteer at one of these events. Working on a committee makes it easy to meet other vegans. Some organizations sponsor weekend or weeklong gatherings. For example, the North American Vegetarian Society (NAVS) holds Vegetarian Summerfest each year (see Appendix A for contact information).

Vegan Communities Online

From *Facebook* to vegan blogs, there are many opportunities to connect with other vegans online. Look for links on your favorite vegan websites or ask friends for suggestions. You can participate as much or as little as you choose.

Vegan Parent Groups

Some larger cities have vegan parent groups. Often these groups are a combination play group/support group. Ask around and check bulletin boards and newspaper calendar listings. The Vegetarian Resource Group (VRG) also has a *Facebook* group for parents (including parents-to-be) who are raising a vegetarian or vegan child. To learn more, go to their website (www.vrg.org).

Will the Baby Be Raised Vegan?

Whether you and your partner are both vegans or you're the only vegan in the house, relatives and friends are likely to wonder how your child will be raised. Chances are if you and your partner are vegan, your baby will be raised as a vegan. Friends may challenge you for not giving your child a choice. Realistically, however, there are many decisions you make for your child—from what religion he practices to where he goes to preschool. When your child is old enough to accept responsibility for these types of decisions, they will be his to make. For now, it's up to you.

Nonvegan family members may be concerned that they won't be able to feed or care for a vegan child. Help them understand that you'll work with them to figure out solutions so they can pamper their vegan grandchild, niece, or nephew.

It gets tricky when one partner is vegan and one is not. You'll learn a lot about each other and about your relationship as you begin to discuss dietary choices for your child. Whether you choose to raise your child vegan, omnivore, vegan at home and nonvegan out of the home, or in some other fashion, the mutual love and respect that brought you together will help you as you assess each option and decide what will work for you.

Getting Help and Support

During or immediately after your pregnancy, you may need help from family or friends. You might be on bed rest or need meals after the baby is born. In an ideal world, you would have dozens of vegan friends and family members who supply your every wish. More realistically, you'll need to work with nonvegans to help them help you.

As a first step, if someone offers to help, be clear about what you can't eat; don't expect people to know what vegan means. Provide recipe ideas and maybe even ingredients. Supplying a carton of soy milk, some vegan margarine, and your favorite brand of egg replacer can be a blessing to a nonvegan cook.

If your friends ask for menu suggestions, keep their food preparation skills in mind. Some people may be more comfortable with simple dishes like beans and rice, pasta salads, and lentil soup. Some friends may enjoy the challenge of using a vegan cookbook that you recommend. Some friends would be happy to pick up takeout, purchase prepared foods that meet your needs, or supply side dishes.

If you have time and energy, you can be proactive. Before the baby is born, make a double batch of some of your favorite recipes—one batch to eat right away and one to freeze for later. Doing this once or twice a week during the last trimester can give you several weeks' worth of vegan meals for when you and your partner want to focus on the baby and not on cooking.

Part 4

Trimester by Trimester

Chapter 12

The First Trimester

During the first trimester, which lasts approximately fourteen weeks from the start of your last period, your baby's growth is amazing. By the end of your first month of pregnancy (four weeks since conception), your child's size will have increased ten-thousandfold. In the second month, your baby will grow from about the size of a raisin to almost the size of a grape. In the next month, your baby will grow to over three inches long and weigh almost 1 ounce, about the size of a roll of Life Savers.

Your Body This Trimester

From the first weeks where you may not notice much more than the absence of your monthly menstrual period to the end of the third month where you have a small potbelly, this first trimester is one of changes. By the end of this trimester, you will definitely feel pregnant. Your body is beginning to make the adjustments that are necessary to support your growing baby. From your tired and anxious mind to your busy bladder, all of your body's systems may seem to be in overdrive during the early days of pregnancy. Stay calm; all of these changes are normal and will become almost second nature as you progress through your pregnancy. It's an exciting time, too, especially at the end of this trimester, when you can hear your baby's heartbeat and perhaps even see him on ultrasound.

Your Body Changes

At the start of your pregnancy, you might not notice any immediate changes in your shape and size. The first thing you will notice is the absence of your monthly menstrual period—in many cases, this is what tipped you off to your pregnancy in the first place. Although you aren't menstruating, you feel slightly bloated, and your waistband may begin to feel a bit snug. On average, most women gain 1–4 pounds in the first trimester.

Some women experience minor vaginal blood flow or spotting as the embryo implants itself into the uterine wall. Because of the timing—one week to ten days after ovulation—it's often mistaken for the beginning of the menstrual period. The spotting, which usually lasts only a day or two, is pink to brown and may be accompanied by minor cramps.

Your breasts may also start to increase in size, and the areolas around your nipples may enlarge and darken. No period? Bigger breasts? This baby is doing wonders for you already! Now for the cloud around that silver lining—fuller breasts are often more tender in pregnancy. A supportive sports bra can help.

You may also experience increased vaginal secretions similar to those you get premenstrually, another hormonal side effect. These typically last throughout pregnancy and may actually worsen in the third trimester, so stock up on panty liners now. Normal vaginal secretions in pregnancy are clear to white in color, mucus-like, and both odor- and pain-free. If you experience discharge that is thick; foul smelling; off-color; or accompanied by itching, blood, or pain, contact your healthcare provider immediately to rule out infection or other problems.

More Changes to Expect

Changes in skin and hair are common in pregnancy. For example, hair that was fine and thin may become thick and shiny during pregnancy, and that fabled pregnancy glow may actually be your flawless, blemish-free complexion. On the other end of the spectrum, acne problems and hair breakage and thinning may occur.

Chloasma (also known as *melasma*) may cause a masklike darkening or lightening of your facial skin. Freckles and moles are prone to darkening, as are other pigmented areas of your skin. To minimize chloasma and other hyperpigmentation, use a good sunscreen (SPF 30 or higher) to cover exposed skin when you're out in the sun.

What You Feel Like

Building a baby is hard work, and even though it's early in the process, it isn't unusual to feel tired and run-down right now. If at all possible, try to grab a nap during the day. If that isn't feasible due to a full-time job or young children at home, make an early bedtime a priority. Although it may run contrary to your nature to be sleeping away the daylight hours, thinking of it as a nap time for baby might help. Once you start down the long road of sleepless nights that new motherhood brings, you'll be longing for the days of early bedtimes and frequent naps!

You may also find yourself spending more and more time in the bathroom. You are urinating more frequently due to high levels of progesterone, which relaxes your bladder muscles. Unfortunately, frequent urination is one symptom that will likely remain with you throughout pregnancy as your baby grows and the uterus exerts more and more pressure on your bladder. Your cardiovascular system is undergoing big changes right now as it adjusts to meet baby's growing demand for the oxygen and nutrients your blood is carrying. Circulating pregnancy hormones dilate (or expand) your blood vessels to accommodate an eventual 40–50 percent increase in blood volume. Your cardiac output, a measure of how hard your heart is working to pump blood, increases 30–50 percent, whereas your blood pressure drops. This is why you may find yourself feeling faint. If you feel dizzy or light-headed, sit or lie down on your side as soon as possible. Try not to lie flat on your back, particularly later in pregnancy, since the pressure your uterus places on two of the large blood vessels that help keep oxygen circulating to you and baby will actually make the dizziness worse.

> If episodes of fainting or dizziness persist or are accompanied by abdominal pain or bleeding, contact your healthcare provider immediately. They could be symptoms of ectopic (or tubal) pregnancy, a potentially fatal condition in which implantation occurs outside the endometrial lining of the uterus.

And then there's the most notorious of all pregnancy symptoms—morning sickness. Referred to by clinicians as nausea and vomiting of pregnancy (or NVP), up to 80 percent of women experience one or both of these symptoms at some point in their pregnancy. NVP can happen at any time and strikes with varying intensity. NVP and relief strategies are covered in depth later in this chapter.

Gas may become a source of discomfort and occasional embarrassment as well. Try to identify triggers and cut back on those foods. Beans, cabbage, broccoli, and carbonated drinks are common offenders. To keep problems at bay, try small, frequent snacks instead of large meals.

At the Doctor's Office

Set up your first prenatal care visit as soon as you know you are pregnant. From now through the seventh month, you'll be seeing your provider on a monthly basis (if you are considered high risk, you may have more frequent appointments). If you're seeing a new doctor or midwife, expect your initial visit to be a bit longer than subsequent checkups since you'll be asked to fill out medical history forms and insurance paperwork. Some providers will send you these materials in advance so you can complete them at home. If you still haven't chosen a provider, now is the time to do so.

Your provider will ask questions about your health history and the pregnancy symptoms you have been experiencing. Make sure that you take advantage of this initial appointment to ask about issues that are on your mind as well. In addition to this interview time, you will undergo a thorough physical examination, give a urine sample (the first of many), and have blood drawn for routine lab work. If you haven't had a Pap smear within the last year, your provider may also perform this test. (For more on diagnostic and screening tests, see Chapter 13.)

> Remember, your partner is in this pregnancy too. By all means, bring him or her to the doctor with you. In addition to providing moral support, he or she probably has just as many questions about the baby as you do. Your partner can also help you remember the things your provider tells you that seem to promptly exit your brain as you leave the examining room.

Your provider will probably supply you with educational brochures and pamphlets on prenatal care, nutrition, office policies, and other important issues. There will be a lot of new information to absorb, so don't feel as though you have to study everything on the spot. However, do take everything home so you can read and refer to it later. Start a folder or notebook for keeping pregnancy information together. Add a pad of paper so you can jot down any questions for your provider.

When to Call the Doctor, Day or Night

At your first appointment, your provider may discuss how patient phone calls are handled both during the day and after office hours. Frequently, obstetric practices use a triage system where the receptionist or intake coordinator answers and prioritizes calls and has a nurse, midwife, or physician return them in order of urgency.

If your doctor is in the office and you feel more comfortable speaking with her directly, be sure to make your preference known when you call.

Usually an answering service will pick up after-hours calls and will page the doctor or midwife on duty, who will then return your call. In most group practices, providers usually take turns covering nights and weekends, so you will get a call back from the on-call practitioner. If you aren't given any guidelines for reaching staff after office hours, make sure you ask. Call your doctor immediately if you experience any of the following symptoms:

- Abdominal pain and/or cramping
- Fluid or blood leaking from the vagina
- Abnormal vaginal discharge (foul smelling, green, or yellow)
- Painful urination
- Severe headache
- Impaired vision (spots, blurring)
- Fever over 101°F
- Chills
- Excessive swelling of face and/or body
- Severe and unrelenting vomiting and/or diarrhea

Some women hesitate to pick up the phone for fear they're being oversensitive or a hypochondriac. While a good dose of common sense should be used in contacting your doctor after office hours, in most cases a better-safe-than-sorry approach applies. Learn to trust your instincts; if something just doesn't feel right to you, make the call.

Get the Most Out of Monthly Checkups

Bring along that list of questions that have come to you and your partner since your last visit. Make sure your questions are answered before you leave; although it's nice to be asked if you have any concerns, in the busy atmosphere of an obstetric practice, your provider may occasionally forget. Never feel like you're being pushy or overbearing (remember, you're leading this team). In most cases, he will do what he can to educate you and reduce any anxieties. If he doesn't, it's never too late to find someone who will.

Baby's Heartbeat

Hearing the steady whoosh-whoosh of your baby's heart for the first time is one of the most thrilling and emotional moments of pregnancy. Your chance at first contact happens the third month as your provider checks for the fetal heartbeat using a small Doppler or Doptone ultrasound device. Make sure your partner makes this month's prenatal appointment. You're both in for a treat as you begin to experience the sights and sounds of your growing child.

On Your Mind

Pregnancy, particularly a first pregnancy, is a time of great anticipation as you head into uncharted waters. Pregnancy is also a precursor to one of the biggest life-changing events there is—the arrival of a baby—and that alone is enough to stir up new and unexpected feelings.

Now that you've officially started this journey, you may be surprised to find yourself filled with conflicting emotions.

Elation, Excitement, and Anxiety

You may be thrilled beyond belief! After all, you are creating a new and unique life of boundless potential. As a family, you will share your hopes, dreams, knowledge, and love. This is one of the most important tasks—and special experiences—of your life. So excitement is the order of the day.

Coupled with the excitement are concerns, of course. You may worry about the baby's health and the possibility of miscarriage early in pregnancy. If you've had a previous miscarriage, you may be walking on eggshells trying to second-guess every move you make. The good news is that knowing your history of miscarriage, your provider is following your progress closely.

Although easier said than done, letting go of your anxieties is the best thing for you and your baby right now. Try designating a certain area of your home, like your bedroom, a worry-free zone, and then stick to a vow to let your anxieties go when you are in that space. Use sounds, sights, and smells to make it as comfortable and relaxing as possible. An aromatherapy candle you like, soft music or nature sounds, and some soothing scenery in the form of photographs and posters can do wonders for your state of mind.

You might also be concerned about your ability to provide for and care for your child. It's important to remember that good parents learn with experience and by the experiences of others. The very fact that you're reading this book and getting regular prenatal care shows that you want the best for your baby. By the time your baby arrives, you'll be surprised at how much you will have learned in the relatively short period of nine months.

Emotional Health

The hormonal changes that occur in pregnancy can have you feeling weepy one minute, irritable the next, and elated thereafter. If you're normally the even-keeled type, these emotional flip-flops can be downright alarming. You aren't losing control or losing your mind; you're just experiencing the normal mood swings of pregnancy. Although this emotional liability may continue throughout pregnancy, it is typically strongest in the first trimester as you adjust to hormonal and other changes.

Stress and Stress Management

It's easy to get stressed out over what may seem like an overwhelming amount of preparation for your new family member. Your body is already working overtime on the development of your child; try to keep your commitments and activities at a reasonable level to prevent mental and physical overload.

Controlling outer stress is especially important when your pregnant body is under the physical stress of providing for a growing baby. And added psychological stress can make the discomforts of pregnancy last longer and feel more severe.

Effective stress management involves finding the right technique for you. Relaxation and meditation techniques (for example, progressive muscle relaxation, yoga); adjustments to your work or social schedule; or carving out an hour of "me time" each evening to decompress are all ways you can lighten your load. Exercise is also a great stress-control method, but be sure to get your doctor's approval regarding the level of exercise appropriate for you.

Forgetfulness

Have you walked around looking for your sunglasses for twenty minutes before finding them on your head? Like any mom-to-be, you've got a lot on your mind. That alone may have you misplacing items and forgetting details that used to be second nature. Although researchers have looked at the problem of memory impairment in pregnancy, there hasn't been a clear consensus on the definitive cause. Pregnancy hormones, sleep deprivation, and stress have all been suggested as possible culprits. Think about carrying a small notebook with you as a memory crutch. This can keep you from losing your mind—and your car.

Morning Sickness

Your stomach flutters, then lurches. Then you run for the bathroom for the fifth time in one morning. Sound like you? NVP is arguably the most debilitating and prevalent of pregnancy symptoms. While most women find that NVP symptoms subside or stop as the first trimester ends, for some they continue into the second and even third trimester. If you're having twins or more, your NVP may also be longer and more intense.

The exact cause of NVP has not been pinpointed, but there are plenty of theories as to why it happens. Some possible culprits: the human chorionic gonadotropin (HCG) hormone that surges through your system and peaks in early pregnancy, a deficiency of vitamin B_6, hormonal changes that relax your gastrointestinal tract and slow digestion, and immune-system changes. Another hypothesis is that morning sickness is actually a defense mechanism that protects both mother and child from toxins and potentially harmful microorganisms in food. No matter what the trigger, it's a miserable time for all.

Remedies and Safety

The following treatments have met with some success in lessening symptoms of NVP in clinical trials. Speak with your healthcare provider before adding any new supplements to your diet.

- Ginger. Gingersnaps and other foods and teas that contain ginger may be helpful in settling your stomach.
- Acupressure wristbands (Sea-Bands). Sometimes used to ward off motion sickness and seasickness, these wristbands place pressure on the P6, or Nei Guan, acupressure point. Available at most drugstores, these bands are an inexpensive and noninvasive way to treat NVP.
- Vitamin B_6. This supplement has reduced NVP symptoms in several clinical trials. It has been suggested that NVP is a sign of vitamin B_6 deficiency.

> Kava kava, licorice root, rue, Chinese cinnamon, and safflower are just a few of the many botanical remedies known to be dangerous in pregnancy. Don't pick up that supplement or cup of herbal tea without asking your healthcare provider first.

Other coping methods that women report as helpful include:

- Eating smaller, more frequent meals. An empty stomach produces acid that can make you feel worse. Low blood sugar causes nausea as well.
- Choosing proteins and complex carbohydrates. Protein-rich foods (tofu, beans) and complex carbs (baked potato, whole-grain breads) are good for the two of you and may calm your stomach.
- Eating what you like. Most pregnant women have at least one food aversion. If broccoli turns your stomach, don't force it. The better foods look and taste, the more likely they are to stay down.
- Sticking to bland foods if you find fatty or spicy foods distasteful. Traditional comfort foods nourish many women suffering through morning sickness; staples like noodle soup, plain rice and pasta, and baked or mashed potatoes can be a filling way to get needed calories.
- Drinking plenty of fluids. Don't get dehydrated. If you're vomiting, you need to replace those lost fluids. Some women report better tolerance of beverages if they are taken between meals rather than with them. Turned off by water and juice right now? Try juicy fruits like watermelon and grapes instead or make your own juice bars by freezing fruit juice in a mold.
- Brushing regularly. Keeping your mouth fresh can cut down on the excess saliva that plagues some pregnant women. Breath mints may be helpful too.

- Asking for help. Preparing meals when you're not feeling well can be even more challenging than eating them, so try to get help in the kitchen from your spouse or significant other, if possible. If not, stock up on foods that require minimal prep work, such as frozen entrées and canned soups, so you can eat with little effort.
- Talking to your provider about switching prenatal vitamins. If it makes you sick just to look at your vitamin, perhaps a chewable or other formulation will help. Iron is notoriously tough on the stomach, so your provider might also recommend a supplement with a lower or extended-release amount. And if you can't keep your vitamin down no matter what you try, your doctor may suggest foregoing it for now until your NVP has passed.

When It May Be More Than Morning Sickness

When your body can't get what it needs from food to keep things running, it will start to metabolize stored fat for energy. This condition, called *ketosis*, generates substances called *ketones* that circulate in your bloodstream and can be harmful to your fetus. Your provider may test your urine for ketones if you're having severe and persistent nausea and vomiting.

Put together a morning sickness survival kit for the car. Items to include: wet wipes, tissues, small bottle of water, travel-sized toothbrush and toothpaste, breath mints, graham or soda crackers, and a bundle of large freezer-grade zip-top baggies. For longer trips, a cell phone and a just-in-case change of clothes are a necessity.

A small percentage of pregnant women (0.3–3 percent) experience a severe form of morning sickness called *hyperemesis gravidarum*. If you can't keep any food or fluids down, are losing weight, and are finding it impossible to function normally, you may be in this category.

Even though hospitalization is sometimes required for hyperemesis gravidarum, the good news is that the treatment—intravenous fluids to restore fluid and electrolyte balance and, in some cases, antiemetics (drugs to stop vomiting)—is relatively simple. If you are prescribed antiemetics, talk with your doctor about the safety data on the drug you are prescribed and any potential effects on the fetus.

If you're dealing with morning sickness, eating healthfully (and keeping it down) is a particular challenge. Your stomach will have definite opinions on what it will and will not tolerate; when you're feeling nauseated, let it guide you. Stick to what works—even if it's the same thing three times daily. Morning sickness won't last forever, and prenatal vitamins will help even out your nutrient intake while you get through this difficult period. Don't worry if you don't gain weight in the first trimester due to morning sickness; it's more important to have weight gain in the following trimesters.

Chapter 13

The Second Trimester

Welcome to the second trimester, what many women consider "the fun part." Your energy is up and your meals are staying down. You're looking pregnant, so take advantage of designated pregnancy parking spaces without feeling guilty. You and your baby are in the midst of a period of rapid growth now, so it's not surprising that you're feeling tired—pregnancy is hard work! Treat yourself to naps and sleeping in on the weekend. Remember, at the end of this trimester, you'll be more than halfway there!

Your Body This Trimester

At the beginning of this trimester, you'll probably actually sense your child inside of you—a humbling and life affirming experience. By the end of the trimester, you may be seeing fetal movement across your abdomen as baby gets comfortable in her shrinking living space. As your uterus expands, your center of gravity shifts, so be careful if you're walking in slippery or icy conditions.

Your appetite is likely to pick up early in the second trimester as well. That's fortunate because you'll gain about 60 percent of your total pregnancy weight (11–15 pounds) in this trimester.

Movement!

Think that ultrasound was exciting? Just wait until you feel your little gymnast stretch and push inside of you for the first time. By week nineteen, most women have felt that distinctive first flutter, often described in terms of butterfly wings or bubbles.

> Once baby starts moving regularly, on average, you should feel five or more movements each hour. Three or fewer movements or a sudden decrease in fetal activity could be a sign of fetal distress, so if you notice either, call your provider to follow up as soon as possible.

You'll quickly discover that your baby is already establishing behavioral patterns. When you're up and about, she can be rocked to sleep by your movements. Then when you lie down and try to take a rest, she wants to get up and groove. Is your partner having trouble getting a hand on your stomach in time to feel the fetal kung fu? Have him or her stand by during a lying-down time to try to catch a kick or two.

Stretch Marks

The skin of your belly is stretching, tightening, and most likely itching like crazy. A good moisturizing cream (look for one that does not contain animal products and that was not tested on animals) can relieve the itching and keep your skin hydrated, although it won't prevent or eliminate stretch marks. Whether or not you develop stretch marks is largely a matter of genetics, although factors such as excessive weight gain and multiples' gestations increase your odds of having them.

> Increased blood volume in pregnancy can damage the valves that regulate blood flow up through the blood vessels of the legs. The result is pooled blood in the vein and that telltale squiggly red or blue line. Supportive stockings and resting on your left side can relieve any leg soreness.

The red, purple, or whitish striae are created by the excess collagen your body produces in response to rapid stretching of the skin. They may appear on your abdomen, breasts, or on any other blossoming body part right now. Don't be too alarmed; striae typically fade to virtually invisible silver lines after pregnancy.

Aches and Pains

You may start to feel occasional discomfort in your lower abdomen, inner thighs, hips, and lower back. A combination of the increased work muscles in these areas are doing and hormonal effects lead to these aches. Pelvic tilt exercises are useful for relieving aches.

The pelvic tilt can be performed while standing against a wall, although it might be more comfortable done on hands and knees. Keep your head aligned with your spine, pull in your abdomen, tighten your buttocks, and tilt your pelvis forward. Your back will naturally arch up. Hold the position for three seconds, and then relax. Remember to keep your back straight in this neutral position. Repeat the tilt three to five times, eventually working up to ten repetitions.

To help with lower back pain, practice good posture when sitting or standing. Avoid sudden twists and turns and put the high heels away for now. Some women find that using a low stool to rest their feet on when sitting helps. If you must stand for long periods, alternate resting each foot on a step. Some stretching and flexibility exercises may be in order. Check with your healthcare provider for approval and recommendations; if the pain is troublesome enough or if you have a history of back problems, he may suggest a physical therapist to work with.

> If your abdominal and/or back pains are severe or accompanied by fever, vomiting, vaginal bleeding, or leg numbness, call your healthcare provider immediately. Most minor back pain in pregnancy is completely normal, but in severe cases it can also be a sign of preterm labor, kidney infection, or other medical problems.

You may also notice leg cramps. Stretching out your calf muscles can often quash a cramp. A number of studies have found that magnesium supplements can reduce the incidence of cramps in some women. Check with your healthcare provider to see what she suggests. Dietary sources of magnesium include whole grains, dried beans, soy products, nuts, and leafy greens.

If your leg pain is accompanied by swelling, redness, and skin that is warm to the touch, call your healthcare provider to report your symptoms. You could be experiencing deep vein thrombosis (DVT), a blood clot in your leg that impedes circulation and has the potential to embolize or break off and block a major blood vessel. Pregnant women are more likely to develop DVT than nonpregnant women; however, DVT itself is relatively rare, occurring in fewer than one of every 1,000 pregnancies.

At the Doctor's Office

Beyond the usual weight and measure routine, your doctor may administer a glucose challenge test (GCT) between weeks twenty-four and twenty-eight. Women who have chosen to take an alpha-fetoprotein (AFP), triple screen, or quad screen test will have their blood drawn sometime between weeks fifteen and eighteen. You can read more about these tests later in this chapter.

Premature Labor

Delivery of your baby after week twenty and before week thirty-seven of pregnancy is considered preterm or premature. In cases of very early preterm labor where fetal lung maturity hasn't been established, your provider will probably try to delay the delivery for as long as possible. Preemies can suffer from a wide range of physical, neurological, and developmental difficulties, so any extra time spent in the womb is beneficial.

If you experience any of the following warning signs of preterm labor, call your healthcare provider immediately. If you are out of town or unable to get in touch with her for any reason, go directly to the nearest hospital emergency room. With prompt action, it may be possible to delay your labor until your unborn child has adequate time to develop.

Symptoms include:

- Painful contractions at regular intervals
- Abdominal cramps
- Lower backache
- Bloody vaginal discharge
- Stomach pain
- Any type of fluid leak from the vagina, large or small

Preterm labor may be halted by bed rest, drugs that stop contractions, and intravenous hydration. Depending on your medical history and the stage of your pregnancy, you may be hospitalized. Home bed rest may also be prescribed, and you might be required to hook up to a fetal monitor on a regular basis. If preterm labor occurs between twenty-four and thirty-four weeks, corticosteroids may be administered to hasten fetal lung development as well.

On Your Mind

It may seem as if you're on an emotional roller coaster. One day you're ready to conquer the world, and the next you feel irritable and overwhelmed. Your emotions are very close to the surface. Try to defuse difficult situations by having an action plan for coping. And don't hesitate to accept small favors such as a closer parking space or a cushy chair in the conference room.

Irritability

Because of all the added demands on your body, mind, and emotional equilibrium, you could be finding yourself short on patience these days. Pregnancy is the perfect excuse for steering clear of people who—let's face it—are just plain annoying. Avoidance isn't the ultimate answer, of course, but during this crucial time in which your emotional and physical balance are so important, it's a good solution for taking care of the little things and keeping your sanity intact.

Definitely continue to buckle up for safety throughout your pregnancy. The lap belt should fit snugly under your belly bulge, and the shoulder belt should be positioned between your breasts. Don't worry about the belt hurting the baby; the uterus and fluid-filled amniotic sac are excellent shock absorbers.

If family and friends are getting your ire up as well, it might be a sign that you are feeling overwhelmed and under supported. Take a look at what's really getting to you. Remember that you aren't in this alone. If you're single, enlist family or close friends to help out. And if you are married or in a relationship but still aren't getting the help and support you need from your partner, ask for it. Although it's nice when others anticipate your needs and pitch in voluntarily, they may be wrapped up in their own preparations and anxieties about the new family addition. Don't feel guilty about reminding them that their help is needed.

Getting Enough Sleep

Perhaps it's nature's way of preparing you for the sleepless nights to come, but your growing belly and the pushes and prods of your little one are making it increasingly difficult to get the requisite eight or more hours of peaceful slumber. Sleep is essential to your mental and physical fitness right now, not to mention that of your unborn child. Make your best effort to rest often and rest well.

- Make a regular bedtime and stick to it.
- If your schedule permits, try to make up your sleep deficit with a daytime nap.
- Experiment with a foam egg-crate cushion on your mattress or a body pillow for extra padding.
- Make the bathroom the last stop before bed.
- Stay away from caffeine (it isn't the best thing for you right now anyway).
- Don't exercise for up to three hours before bedtime.

Exercise

Don't avoid the gym, pool, or other favorite places to exercise just because you're pregnant. Exercise will not only make you feel better; it can tone muscles that will be getting a workout in labor and delivery.

> Certain activities are definitely off-limits during pregnancy. These include scuba diving, water skiing, downhill snow skiing, and contact sports. Gymnastics and horseback riding should be avoided because of the increased risk of falling. In addition, proceed with caution when participating in potentially high-impact activities like tennis, volleyball, and aerobics.

Exercise guidelines issued by ACOG recommend twenty to thirty minutes of moderate exercise activity daily for women who are pregnant (excluding high-risk pregnancies), or about 150 minutes per week. Swimming and walking are examples of recommended forms of exercise. More-strenuous exercise (like jogging and some sports) may be fine during pregnancy if you are physically fit and exercised before you were pregnant. All pregnant women, especially those in high-risk pregnancies and those who were inactive prior to pregnancy, should speak with their physician about exercise options.

Exercise doesn't have to be complicated, expensive, or technically difficult. It can be as simple as tossing a ball with the kids in the backyard, taking the dog on a brisk walk each evening, or swimming or even walking laps in the local pool.

Thirty minutes of regular, heart-pumping activity started and capped off by a good stretching routine is all it takes to benefit you and baby. Above all, make sure it's an activity you enjoy or do in good company so you will look forward to it.

If you thrive on routine and feel more likely to get moving if you have a set schedule, check out your local YMCA, hospital, or community center for a prenatal exercise class. Water exercise programs are also a good low-impact way to get fit. Even if your class is tailored toward moms-to-be, check with your doctor first.

Precautions

While exercise can be a boon to your body and baby, there are basic steps you should take to stay safe. First and foremost, run your routine by your provider to get a medical stamp of approval. If you're new to working out, start slowly. Be attuned to your body's signals and stop immediately if you experience warning signs such as abdominal or chest pain, vaginal bleeding, dizziness, blurred vision, severe headache, or excessive shortness of breath.

Dress in supportive, comfortable clothing that breathes well and braces your belly and other parts of your expanding anatomy. If your feet have swollen past the comfort level of your old gym shoes, invest in a bigger pair. Drink plenty of caffeine-free fluids before, during, and after your workout to remain well hydrated, and try to work out in a climate-controlled environment to avoid a sharp rise in core body temperature since overheating can be hazardous to a developing fetus.

Kegels are one exercise every pregnant woman should know and practice. They strengthen the pelvic muscles for delivery and can improve the urinary incontinence (or dribbling) that some women experience in pregnancy. What are Kegels? Tighten the muscles you use to shut off your urine flow, hold for four seconds, and relax. You've just done your first Kegel. Try to work up to ten minutes of Kegels daily.

Screening and Diagnostic Tests

You'll be poked, prodded, swabbed, scraped, and scanned throughout your pregnancy. All these tests have a purpose, of course—a healthy mom and baby. Prenatal tests elicit the full spectrum of maternal emotions, from calm reassurance to amusement to anxiety and fear of the unknown. Knowing what to expect can make these exams more comfortable.

Urine Tests

You'll be giving a urine sample at each prenatal visit for urinalysis. Your provider's office or lab will test your urine for ketones, protein, and glucose, and may also check for the presence of any bacteria. These tests are simple; a strip of chemically treated paper is dipped in your urine sample. Your urine is tested for ketones as indicators of either insufficient nourishment due to severe nausea and vomiting or poorly controlled gestational diabetes. The test for protein in your urine is a check for preeclampsia, urinary tract infection (UTI), and renal (kidney) impairment. Glucose (or sugar) in the urine (called *glycosuria*) can be a sign of gestational diabetes mellitus (GDM). It's normal to spill a small amount of sugar into the urine in pregnancy, but consistently high levels along with other risk factors raise a red flag that GDM may be present. Positive results on any of these tests usually call for additional testing.

Blood Work

Early in pregnancy, and possibly in the second and third trimesters, your blood hemoglobin level will be measured to check for iron-deficiency anemia. Blood tests can also screen for inherited anemia in at-risk populations. For example, couples of African, Caribbean, Eastern Mediterranean, Middle Eastern, and Asian descent are at risk for sickle cell anemia. Families of Greek, Italian, Turkish, African, West Indian, Arab, or Asian descent may be screened for the thalassemia trait.

Your blood type and Rhesus (or Rh) factor will be determined at your first prenatal visit. An Rh factor is either positive or negative. If your Rh is positive, no treatment is necessary. If you are Rh negative and your partner is Rh positive, you are at risk for Rh incompatibility with the blood type of your baby. Rh incompatibility can occur when your unborn baby is Rh positive. If some of the baby's blood enters your bloodstream, your body may produce antibodies against the baby's blood, causing her to have severe anemia. When this happens, your immune system may try to fight off the baby as an intruder, causing serious complications. If caught early on, however, the disorder can be treated effectively later in pregnancy.

Blood tests also determine whether or not you are immune to German measles (rubella), a disease that can cause birth defects, especially if you contract it during the first trimester. An HIV, hepatitis B, and syphilis test may also be done on your blood.

Women over age thirty-five have a higher risk for developing diabetes, high blood pressure, and placental problems in pregnancy. There is also an increased risk of having a baby with a chromosomal disorder. The good news is that proper prenatal care can greatly reduce your risk of these complications.

Typically between weeks twenty-four and twenty-eight of pregnancy, you will be given a glucose challenge test as a screening tool for GDM. The test requires you to drink 50 grams of a glucose solution, a sugary flavored drink usually called *Glucola*. One hour later, blood will be drawn, and your blood glucose levels will be measured. If your results exceed the guidelines your doctor has established, further testing will be necessary.

Swabs and Smears

Unless you've had one in the twelve months leading up to conception, your provider will give you a Pap smear at your initial prenatal visit. Swabs of both the rectum and the vagina will be done at weeks thirty-five through thirty-seven of gestation to check for Group B streptococcus (GBS). If a pregnant woman tests positive for this bacterium that can cause serious infections in a newborn, she is usually prescribed intravenous antibiotics during labor and delivery. Depending on your medical history and perceived risk factors, your provider may also test for chlamydia, gonorrhea, or bacterial vaginosis by means of a vaginal swab sample.

Ultrasounds

The eagerly awaited ultrasound gives you your first glimpse at your little one and lets your practitioner assess the baby's growth and development. It may also be used to diagnose placental abnormalities, an ectopic pregnancy, certain birth defects, or other suspected problems. There are two types of ultrasound scans: the transabdominal, which scans through your abdomen, and the transvaginal, which scans directly into your vagina. In very early pregnancy, the technician may opt for the vaginal approach, which means that the transducer (or handheld wand) will be inserted into your vagina. However, abdominal ultrasounds are the most common since most ultrasounds take place in the second or third trimesters.

> If your fetus isn't feeling coy on ultrasound day, a sonogram taken after sixteen weeks may reveal its sex. A sighting of a girl's labia (visible as three parallel lines) or a boy's penis can provide a fairly positive ID, but keep in mind that ultrasound is not foolproof and parents have been surprised in the delivery room.

An ultrasound typically takes no longer than a half hour to perform. If you are in the first half of your pregnancy, you will probably be instructed to drink plenty of water prior to the exam and refrain from emptying your bladder. This is probably the most difficult part of the test. The extra fluids help the technician visualize your baby.

Many obstetricians order ultrasounds as a matter of routine. Some do one at the first visit to check for correct dates and viability, with the rationale that it may save them from questioning gestational dates later on (since dating is more accurate when done in the first trimester). Others will recommend a sonogram at around week twenty to examine the fetal anatomy and ensure the pregnancy is progressing normally.

AFP, Triple Screen, and Quad Screen Tests and Cell-Free DNA

The maternal serum AFP test, usually administered between weeks fifteen and eighteen, is a blood test used to screen for chromosomal irregularities such as trisomy 18 and trisomy 21 (Down syndrome), and also for neural tube defects. It can also indicate the presence of twins, triplets, or more. A more precise version of the AFP test is the triple screen test (or AFP-3), which measures levels of HCG and estriol, a type of estrogen, as well as AFP. The quad screen test, an even more sensitive marker of chromosomal problems, assesses all three of these substances plus inhibin A.

You may also hear about noninvasive prenatal testing (NIPT). This is becoming an increasingly popular choice in testing in the United States. In fact, some obstetricians now standardly offer cell-free DNA (cfDNA) testing to all high-risk patients. While this option is more expensive than quad screen testing, recent studies like those covered in *The New England Journal of Medicine* found that cfDNA testing had significantly lower false positive rates and higher positive predictive values for trisomy 18 and 21.

Amniocentesis

An amniocentesis, or amnio, involves two critical undertakings: a needle being inserted through the abdomen and breeching your baby's watery environment. It does carry some risk of complications, including a slight chance of miscarriage. However, the amnio is one of the best tools available for diagnosing genetic disorders and chromosomal abnormalities. An amnio is typically performed in the second trimester sometime between weeks fifteen and twenty of pregnancy, although a later amnio may be done depending on the indication.

> The CDC estimates the chance of miscarriage following an amnio at somewhere between 1 in 400 and 1 in 200, and the risk of uterine infection at less than 1 in 1,000. There is also a slight risk of trauma to the unborn baby from a misplaced needle or inadvertent rupture of the sac.

Your provider may suggest you meet with a genetic counselor prior to having an amniocentesis performed to weigh the risks versus the benefits of the procedure, given your specific medical background and family history.

After the amnio procedure, the baby will be monitored by ultrasound and will have his heart rate checked for a few minutes to ensure that everything is okay. Minimal cramping may follow the procedure. You will be advised to restrict strenuous exercise for a day (no step aerobics and no sex), although other normal activity should be fine. If in the days following the amnio you experience fluid or blood discharge from the vagina, let your provider know as soon as possible.

Chorionic Villus Sampling (CVS)

CVS is performed in the first trimester (usually between weeks ten and twelve) to assess chromosomal abnormalities and hereditary conditions in the unborn baby. Your provider will use ultrasound guidance to insert a catheter into the placenta, either through the cervix or through a needle injected into the abdomen. The catheter is used to extract a biopsy (or sample) of the tiny chorionic villi, the fingers of tissue surrounding the embryo that are the beginnings of the placenta. The villi are a genetic match for the baby's own tissue.

Slight cramping and spotting is normal after the procedure, and you will probably be advised to indulge in some rest and relaxation for the remainder of the day. If bleeding continues, is excessive, or is accompanied by pain or fever, call your practitioner immediately.

> Some studies suggest that the experience and associated skill level of the physician performing a CVS or amniocentesis can make a big difference in the risk of complications. Many physicians will refer you to a specialist for just this reason. If your provider is performing the procedure, ask for an estimate of how many amnios or CVS procedures he has performed.

CVS has several benefits over amnio. It can be performed earlier (first trimester as opposed to second), and the results are available much faster (five to seven days for preliminary CVS results versus ten to fourteen days for amnio). However, the risk of miscarriage is higher with CVS—between 1 in 200 and 1 in 100 will experience miscarriage after the procedure. The risk is higher for women with a retroverted (tipped or tilted) uterus who are given a transcervical CVS (about 5 in 100 according to the National Health Service in the UK). For this reason, a transabdominal CVS (through the abdominal wall) is usually advised for these women. A consultation with a genetic counselor can help you analyze the positives and negatives and decide whether a CVS is right for you.

Fetal Monitoring

A fetal heart monitor measures the fetal heart rate (or FHR). A baseline (or average) fetal heart rate of 120–160 beats per minute (bpm) is considered normal. During your routine prenatal exams, a handheld monitor is used to quickly listen to the fetal heart rate. If you need to be monitored for a longer period of time, belts are used to keep the monitors in place for a period of about twenty minutes. When being monitored, your healthcare provider will look for fetal heart rate accelerations, which correspond to your baby's movement and are a sign of fetal well-being. Reasons to have the prolonged monitoring include going past your due date, intrauterine growth restriction (IUGR), GDM, and other medical conditions.

Vegan-Friendly Options for Pregnancy Testing

There are two main diagnostic tests for which you might want to choose vegan-friendly options if possible: a glucose challenge test and an ultrasound.

The Glucose Challenge Test

The glucose challenge test is a test used to detect gestational diabetes. Pregnancy tends to lower a woman's tolerance to glucose by increasing resistance to insulin, the hormone that drives the glucose into the cells. What can result is gestational diabetes mellitus (GDM), which affects anywhere from 2 to 10 percent of pregnancies in the US, according to the CDC.

Obesity is a major risk factor for GDM. Unfortunately, due to the epidemic of obesity in our country, it is on the rise. GDM increases the risk for high blood pressure, a large baby, and premature birth. It increases the risk for type 2 diabetes in the mother (50 percent) later in life and in the child (as he or she grows) as well. That is why it is important to be tested.

Your doctor will suggest you have the test performed between weeks twenty-four and twenty-eight. Typically, you will be given a drink called *Glucola*. You eat a normal meal beforehand. Then you drink the solution, which contains 50 grams of sugar. One hour later your blood sugar is checked by a blood draw. If your sugar is 130–140 mg/dl or higher, you will go on to complete a glucose tolerance test. This involves drinking 75 grams of sugar for a two-hour test or 100 grams of sugar for a three-hour test.

In 2016, the US Preventive Services Task Force did a meta-analysis utilizing fifteen databases and found the challenge test to be quite sensitive for picking up GDM. It confirmed that the 50-gram Glucola test was an effective screening tool. The question is how safe is Glucola? And, is it vegan? It is (most likely) vegan; however, some of the stuff it contains has raised the hackles of many.

The drink contains dextrose that is typically vegan, but it may be filtered through bone char filtration. It also contains citric acid and sodium benzoate, both vegan. There are two food coloring dyes used: yellow #6 and red #40. The yellow dye is vegan but is still food coloring, and the red dye comes from coal. There is natural flavoring, and there is no way to tell where this comes from. The drink tastes pretty nasty and can cause nausea and dizziness.

Is there an alternative? Possibly. However, are the alternatives as good as Glucola for detecting GDM?

In 1999, researchers substituted twenty-eight jelly beans for Glucola. The test results were similar, and there were fewer side effects with the jelly beans.

If the challenge test is positive, more jelly beans can be used to increase the amount of sugar given (75 or 100 grams) in order to administer the glucose tolerance test, according to a 1999 article in the *American Journal of Obstetrics & Gynecology*.

A study done in 2013 found that ten Twizzlers Strawberry Twists were as good at detecting diabetes as the 50-gram Glucola drink. This test was done in nonpregnant subjects initially. In 2015, it was found to be effective in pregnant subjects as well. There were fewer side effects and false positive tests.

Twizzlers Strawberry Twists are both vegan and kosher. They do contain red dye that is approved by the FDA and high fructose corn syrup. If that is a problem for you, organically flavored jelly beans may be a better choice.

Ultrasound

For an ultrasound, a gel will be placed on the skin to help a transducer pass over your belly, using sound waves to examine your baby in utero. It can detect the heartbeat and find potential issues that might affect the outcome of your pregnancy. The standard gel contains the following:

- Propylene glycol: an organic oil.
- Glycerin: a polyol compound used in gels that absorbs water from air.
- Phenoxyethanol: a glycol ether. It has a warning from the FDA in 2008 of being potentially toxic and can damage the nervous system.
- Colorant: typically blue for ultrasound gels.

These ingredients are vegan but contain chemicals. There is a new ultrasound gel (just released in 2018) called *EcoVue*. It contains no parabens or propylene glycol. It is eco-friendly, vegan, and kosher, and it uses fermented natural products. Since it is a relatively new product, you may have to ask your ultrasonographer about it.

These are the two major tests that most women will have during pregnancy, and there are ways they can be more pleasant and natural. Find a nonconfrontational way to ask your provider about them.

Common Concerns: Heartburn and Hemorrhoids

Sometime in the second trimester, you may begin to experience heartburn, a burning feeling in your chest or throat. This feeling is due to stomach acid moving up into your esophagus. It's not uncommon in pregnancy and is due to your uterus crowding your stomach. Hormonal changes also have an effect by making muscles in your digestive tract remain relaxed rather than tightening to block acid movement out of the stomach.

There are some ways to reduce heartburn:

- Stay away from alcohol and caffeinated drinks; these can relax the valve between the stomach and the esophagus and exacerbate heartburn.
- Keep a food log to determine your heartburn triggers; many women find it helps to avoid greasy or spicy foods.

- Eat smaller, more frequent meals instead of three large ones.
- Don't eat just before you go to bed or lie down to rest.
- Rest your head on a few extra pillows in bed to assist gravity in easing heartburn while you sleep.

If heartburn symptoms won't relent, there are several over-the-counter antacids and medications available considered safe to use in pregnancy. Speak with your doctor to find the one right for you.

Being a vegan may help you avoid symptoms of another common condition: hemorrhoids. Hemorrhoids are swollen, inflamed veins around the anus or lower rectum. They can become itchy, painful, and perhaps even protrude from the anus. These swollen veins are caused by increased pressure from your growing uterus on the rectal veins coupled with pregnancy hormones that can cause veins to dilate and swell. When you strain to have a bowel movement or have a hard bowel movement, the hemorrhoid's fragile surface can be damaged and it can bleed. Vegan diets are typically high in fiber. This high-fiber diet, along with exercise and plenty of water, can help you avoid constipation and straining with bowel movements that may aggravate hemorrhoids. If you do have painful hemorrhoids, try easing the pain with an ice pack, a soak in a warm tub, wipes or pads with witch hazel, or a topical prescription cream as recommended by your doctor.

Chapter 14

The Third Trimester

It's the homestretch, the big countdown—the third trimester. You've made a lot of decisions so far, and there are even more to be made in the next few months. You'll be getting ready for labor and delivery as you sort through your options for childbirth classes and assemble a birth plan. You may feel some Braxton-Hicks contractions (discussed in an upcoming section in this chapter) as your body starts prepping for the hard work of labor. Consider them a dress rehearsal for the big event.

Your Body This Trimester

You're likely feeling perpetually stuffed and slightly out of breath as your uterus relocates all your internal organs. The relief and energy felt in the second trimester can start to fade now. Just remember: you're almost there!

At the beginning of this trimester, the top of the fundus (uterus) is halfway between your belly button and your breastbone, displacing your stomach, intestines, and diaphragm. It's increasingly easy to get winded as your little one pushes up into your diaphragm. Take it slow, breathe deeply, and practice good posture. To ease breathing while you sleep, pile on a few extra pillows or use a foam bed wedge to elevate your head.

Not only are your breasts heavier, but they are more glandular and getting ready to feed your baby. In this last trimester, your nipples may begin to leak colostrum, which is the yellowish, nutrient-rich fluid that precedes real breast milk. You may find the leaking more apparent when you're sexually aroused. To reduce backaches and breast tenderness, make sure you wear a well-fitting bra (even to bed if it helps). If you are planning on breastfeeding, you might want to consider buying some supportive nursing bras now that can take you through the rest of pregnancy and right into the postpartum period.

> If you're picking up nursing bras, be sure to test-drive the clasps for easy access. Try to unfasten and slip the nursing flaps down with one hand. This may seem unimportant now, but when you're in a crowded shopping mall trying to discreetly put baby to breast single-handedly, you'll be thankful you had the foresight.

As baby settles firmly on your bladder, bathroom stops step up once again. You may even experience some stress incontinence, which is minor dribbling or leakage of urine when you sneeze, cough, laugh, or make other sudden movements. This will clear up postpartum. In the meantime, keep doing your Kegels, don't hold it in, and wear a panty liner.

Braxton-Hicks Contractions

This trimester, your body is warming up for labor, and you may start to experience Braxton-Hicks contractions. These painless and irregular contractions feel as if your uterus is making a fist and then gradually relaxing. If your little one is fairly active, you might think that he is stretching himself sideways at first. A quick check of your belly will reveal a visible tightening.

Braxton-Hicks contractions can begin as early as week twenty and continue right up until your due date, although these contractions are more commonly felt in the final month of pregnancy. Some first-time moms-to-be are afraid they won't be able to tell the difference between Braxton-Hicks and actual labor contractions. As any woman who has been through labor can attest, when the real thing comes, you'll know it. Rule of thumb: if it hurts, it's labor.

> The average labor lasts twelve to fourteen hours, plenty of time to get to the hospital. To avoid any unforeseen delays, work out a route in advance, keep your gas tank full, and have cash on hand for a cab in case your car conks out with the first contraction.

If your contractions suddenly seem to be coming at regular intervals and they start to cause you pain or discomfort, they could be the real thing. Lie down on your left side for about a half hour with a clock or watch on hand and time the contractions from the beginning of one to the beginning of the next. If the interludes are more or less regular, call your healthcare provider. And if contractions of any type are accompanied by blood or amniotic fluid leakage, contact your practitioner immediately.

Your Body—Changes in the Last Month

Engagement (or lightening), the process of the baby dropping down into the pelvic cavity in preparation for delivery, can occur anytime now. In some women, particularly those who have given birth before, it may not happen until labor starts.

Your cervix is ripening (softening) in preparation for baby's passage. As it effaces (thins) and dilates (opens), the soft plug of mucus keeping it sealed tight may be dislodged. This mass, which has the appealing name of *mucous plug*, may be tinged red or pink.

If the baby has dropped, you could be running to the bathroom more than ever. She also may be sending shock waves through your pelvis as she settles farther down onto the pelvic floor. An upside is that you can finally breathe more easily as she pulls away from your lungs and diaphragm. Braxton-Hicks contractions can be more frequent this month as you draw nearer to delivery. You're close enough to be on the lookout for the real thing, however. How will you recognize them?

Real contractions will:

- Be felt in the back and possibly radiate around to the abdomen.
- Not subside when you move around or change positions.
- Increase in intensity as time passes.
- Come at roughly regular intervals (early on, this can be from twenty to forty-five minutes apart).
- Increase in intensity with activity like walking.

Other signs that labor is on its way include amniotic fluid that leaks in either a gush or a trickle (your "water breaking"), sudden diarrhea, and the appearance of the mucous plug. Keep in mind, however, that for many women, the bag of waters does not break until active labor sets in.

At the Doctor's Office

This trimester, your visits to the doctor might start to step up to twice monthly, with weekly visits in the last month. Your provider will probably want to know whether you've been experiencing any Braxton-Hicks contractions, and he will cover the warning signs of preterm labor and what you should do if you experience them.

Sometime in your eighth month, your practitioner will check the position of your baby to determine whether she has turned head down in preparation for birth. You may learn that your baby is in breech position (bottom or foot first). Don't panic. Your fickle fetus is likely to change position again in the next few weeks. If she doesn't, your practitioner may try to turn the baby closer to term.

Amniotic fluid is clear to straw-colored and has a faintly sweet smell. Less commonly, it may be tinged green or brown. If you think you're leaking amniotic fluid, no matter how small the amount, contact your care provider. If your membranes have ruptured, you risk infection if you don't deliver soon.

In the last month, unless you are scheduled for a planned cesarean section, your provider will probably perform an internal exam with each visit to check your cervix for changes that indicate approaching labor. She'll also be taking note of any descent or dropping of the baby toward the pelvis. Although you may start effacing and dilating now, it's still anyone's guess as to when labor will begin, and it could be a few more weeks yet.

On Your Mind

As labor looms closer, your thoughts turn to the task at hand. Going into labor and delivery with as much knowledge of the process as possible can make the difference between a positive childbirth experience and a frustrating one.

Am I Up to the Task of Labor?

Women have been doing this since the beginning of time and under much more difficult circumstances. Yes, in most cases labor will be hard work, but if you prepare yourself by learning what to expect, you will be ready to face whatever comes your way. You'll also find that your spouse or labor partner and coach will be a huge asset in helping you through childbirth.

Am I Up to the Task of Motherhood?

Great mommies are made, not born. Although some aspects of mothering will seem to come to you instinctively, practice and trial and error will make up the better part of your parenting education. Use the tools around you—your pediatrician, other parents, and research and reading—to build and sharpen your skills. In the final analysis, listen to your inner voice in the application of what you learn.

Nesting

Nesting is that overwhelming urge to prepare a safe haven for your little one and assure yourself that all his needs and wants will be adequately met. You may be trying to furnish a nursery and clean the house—both instinctive reactions to the upcoming arrival.

Keep in mind that during the first few weeks home, keeping baby within arm's length will improve your rest and peace of mind. A bassinet can make her feel safer and more secure than in the open space of a crib after spending nine months in close quarters. And you can roll a bassinet right next to your bed to give those 4 a.m. feedings with ease.

Some baby essentials you should have on hand prior to his arrival: diapers, wipes, alcohol swabs (for his umbilical cord), vegan baby shampoo and soap, vegan diaper-rash ointment, waterproof pads, bottles, a thermometer, and a fever-reducing product (Tylenol) recommended by your pediatrician.

Don't go crazy buying supersized cases of baby supplies; buy small so you can sample. Once you've decided what works best for you and baby, you can stock up. Now is the time to start thinking about whether you want to go cloth or disposable with diapers. If you're thinking green, cloth diapers have the advantage of not ending up in a landfill, although they do require additional fossil fuels and water resources to wash and transport (if you use a service). Call local diaper services to get estimates and a rundown of what's included. You can wash diapers at home, of course, but be sure you have the time to be doing laundry daily. If your baby has sensitive skin, you might find cloth less irritating. Like most things in parenting, it's trial and error—have a supply of both and see how each works for you.

Setting Up a Vegan Nursery

Most baby supplies, from diaper-rash cream to baby shampoo, are available in vegan versions. Check a well-stocked natural foods store or co-op or look for online vegan supply companies. See Appendix A for some ideas. You may want to start by buying small sizes to see which brands you prefer. Check with other parents on vegetarian or vegan parent email lists to see if there are brands that other parents recommend.

On Your Mind—The Last Month

You are so ready to have this baby. Nothing fits, not even your shoes. You can't sleep for more than a few hours at a time. You look toward your due date like a long-distance runner approaching the end of a marathon. As you waddle toward the finish line, enjoy these final sensations of your child moving inside of you—the funny little hiccups, the elbow and knee bumps parading across your belly, and the subtle nudges that remind you you're not alone even if no one else is around. Relish these final days of exhilaration and anticipation—they are unique.

First-time moms may find themselves overwhelmed with anxiety now that birth is so near. Take a deep breath, go over what you learned in childbirth class, and talk with your partner or labor coach about ways to get past the anxious feelings. It's perfectly natural to be fearful of the unknown, but don't let fear wrest control of your labor from you.

Even if you have been through pregnancy already, you might still be anxious about baby's arrival. Perhaps you're following a different kind of labor and birth plan or you're concerned about how your other child will react to his new sibling. Again, talk it out with your partner, ask your provider any questions that are still on your mind about labor and delivery, and remember that you've been through this once and you'll make it through again.

Childbirth Classes

Most childbirth seminars available through hospitals and birthing centers are called *prepared childbirth classes*. Taking place in a classroom setting and using lectures, audiovisual aids, and floor exercises to get you ready for labor and delivery, prepared childbirth classes usually focus on one, two, or more birth philosophies. They can vary in length from several months of Saturdays to a one-day seminar. While hospital policy will dictate a lot of what's covered, you can expect to get a guided tour of the facility, learn what goes on in labor and delivery, and find out some basics of caring for a new baby. Your spouse, partner, or labor coach will learn more about his or her role in the process. You'll get all sorts of brochures, handouts, and forms that you can read at home. Perhaps the most important facet of childbirth class (and certainly the one that most first-time moms pay the closest attention to) is the information it provides on managing labor and delivery discomforts. In addition to an overview of anesthesia and pain medication options, childbirth educators draw on one or more childbirth philosophies to teach coping methods.

To find out about what's available, call your hospital or birthing center and ask for schedules and descriptions of upcoming classes. Once you get a feel for what is offered, call with follow-up questions about instructor credentials and training, methods taught, class size, curriculum, and costs. You might also ask if there are couples who have taken the course that you can contact as references.

> If you've had a previous cesarean section, ask about a VBAC class, which provides couples with information on the benefits, risks, and statistics surrounding vaginal births following a cesarean section. They are usually recommended as a supplement to, rather than a replacement for, a prepared childbirth class.

Even if you don't choose a childbirth class sponsored by the facility where you'll be giving birth, you should try to arrange a tour. Getting your bearings ahead of time will save you valuable time and frustration when the big day arrives. You'll also have less anxiety if you know what to expect of the labor and birthing rooms.

New-sibling classes can be a huge boon for families with other children. Typically divided by age group so information can be communicated at an appropriate level, these classes put an emphasis on how things at home are changing, how the family will adjust after baby is born, and what the children are feeling about these developments. A sibling class can help your child feel more involved in and, consequently, more accepting of your family's growth.

Writing Your Birth Plan

Are you looking forward to a completely chemical-free birth or are you already exploring your painkilling options? Do you want only your partner in attendance or would you like additional support? Your birth plan is your chance to let everyone involved know what you want the experience to be. Whatever your idea of perfect labor and delivery is, make sure the direction of your birth plan is driven by the needs of your partner and you and not by the expectations of others. Remember, of course, that plans can change as conditions change during labor and delivery. Appendix B in the back of this book includes a checklist you can use for guidance in creating your birth plan. Also take a look at the next chapter, which provides more information about labor and delivery.

Developing a birth plan can ease your anxieties and serve as a springboard for discussions with your partner. Because the plan can tread on some sensitive and controversial medical territory, it's important that your provider be included in the process.

Working with Your Provider

Once you and your partner have your birth plan together, you should present it to your provider for his comments and questions. Communicating your wishes and being receptive to feedback can make the difference between a birth plan that works and one that doesn't.

Consider the plan you initially take to your provider a first draft. Be willing to really listen to any suggestions or issues your provider has and make an effort to work toward a resolution together. Also, try to keep your expectations grounded in reality and not overly restrictive. After your discussion, you can incorporate your provider's input into your final plan.

While covering all your bases is important, you simply can't control every possible aspect of what does or doesn't occur during labor and delivery. Medical emergencies do happen, which is why you have signed on with a practitioner to begin with. You need to trust your provider to follow the spirit of your birth plan while making adjustments for your health and that of your baby. Establishing a good communicative relationship is the best way to ensure this.

Your doctor will warn you up front that unforeseen circumstances will mean a deviation from your birth plan. Sometimes women feel as if they have failed if matters do not go precisely according to their concept of "the ideal birth," which is certainly not realistic. The best way to avoid disappointment is to build alternative scenarios into your birth plan regarding interventions that might be required. For example, if you really don't want an episiotomy, you should indicate that in your birth plan and suggest perineal massage with vitamin E oil or another lubricant, warm compresses, or another acceptable alternative. But be prepared to work with your doctor during labor if your alternative plan just doesn't do the trick.

Some vegans will wonder if medications and supplies used in their treatment are vegan. The Vegan Society in the UK maintains a listing of animal-free medications at www.vegansociety.com/resources/nutrition-and-health/medications/list-animal-free-medications. This list is not comprehensive and may not include medications available in the United States. You can certainly ask your doctor if vegan alternatives are available for commonly used medications (if the medication is supplied in a gelatin-based capsule, it may also be available as a liquid or tablet). You can also discuss your preference for vegan medications and supplies. However, in many cases practitioners simply don't know if medications are vegan or not. Try to do your best, keep in mind that your health and the well-being of your baby are very important, and that your dietary choices are already promoting a more humane world.

Gearing Up for the Big Event

Since baby's timetable is somewhat unpredictable, start getting your affairs in order at the beginning of the ninth month. Cover all personal, professional, and family bases to ensure a smooth transition from home to hospital and back home again. For example, double-check with your provider that a copy of your birth plan has been put into your chart, and verify any changes you might have made to the plan since your first review together.

Being Vegan in the Hospital

Most hospitals, sad to say, don't routinely serve vegan meals. If you'd prefer not to pick at a salad and maybe some steamed vegetables during your stay, some planning ahead of time is key. Start by reminding your doctor that you are vegan so that a vegan diet order can be placed on your chart. Contact the dietary department at the hospital prior to your due date, describe your diet, and ask how they will meet your needs. Ask about bringing some of your own food, especially basics like soy milk. Can your partner supply vegan takeout for a post-delivery celebratory meal? Be sure to find out whom to contact and how to contact them should anything go wrong once you're in the hospital.

Pack Your Bag

You'll probably pack and unpack your bag a half dozen times this month making sure you have everything you could possibly need. Don't go crazy with work or entertainment equipment—you'll be too busy with labor, delivery, and meeting and caring for your child.

Essentials you should have:

- Pain-relief tools and music for labor: things like massage balls, a picture for focusing on through contractions, a water bottle. Check with your hospital or birthing center to see whether a small portable stereo is acceptable. If not, bring personal headphones.
- Snacks for the coach. Make sure it's something that won't turn your stomach during labor.
- A camera. For capturing baby's arrival (or the moments shortly thereafter). Don't forget batteries and an extra memory card!
- Stopwatch or watch with a second hand for timing contractions.
- Clothes for you. Include several nightgowns with button or snap fronts if you're going to nurse, a bathrobe, extra underwear, socks and/or slippers for those cold floors, and something loose and comfortable to wear to go home. And be sure to bring glasses or contacts if you need them.

- Sanitary pads. The hospital will provide you with some, but extras are good to have on hand.
- Phone numbers. Bring names and numbers of the folks you'll want to call immediately.
- Something for siblings. A big sister/brother gift and their photo on the newborn's bassinet can make their introduction smoother.
- Toiletries and shower supplies. Bring your chosen brand of vegan toothpaste, shampoo, and other basics along with a toothbrush.
- A going-home outfit for baby. Pack a set of newborn clothes and a baby blanket. Let your partner bring the car seat on discharge day.

If you're breastfeeding, you might also pack:

- Nursing bras. If you don't have any yet, a bra with a front fastener will work well as a stand-in for now.
- A box of nursing pads for when your milk comes in.
- Vitamin E oil or vegan ointment for sore or cracked nipples.

Recruit Help Now!

Now is the time to take friends, family, and neighbors up on their offers of assistance. If they ask whether they can help, say yes! Make a list and schedule assignments. Give friends who are good in the kitchen ideas for easy vegan meals they can prepare for you. If you have other children, make sure their schedules are covered.

Feel like you need some live-in help to get you through the first week or so? Ask a mommy expert, maybe your own mom, to come for a visit. Sound out the idea with your mate—he or she may feel this is a special family time but might reconsider after hearing your reasons. Just make sure your guest isn't someone who will add to your stress.

Finalize Maternity-Leave Plans

If you're working right up until your due date, start clearing the decks early in the month. Make sure coworkers and managers are regularly apprised of where outstanding projects stand, and try to treat every day as if it might be your last before you leave. The more you enable matters to flow smoothly in your absence, the less likely you are to get calls at home.

Talk with your supervisor about communication during your absence. If you want to remain incommunicado (and you have every right to do so), make your feelings known. You might limit any contact you do agree to, such as emails only or phone calls only in a certain window of time each day. Remember, this is your time off both to recuperate and to get to know your child.

Hurry Up and Wait (When Baby Is Late)

You've finally reached that magic EDD (expected delivery date) and…nothing. Don't be too depressed. Instead, try to stay busy, and if you feel up to it, get out and about. Unless you have a precise twenty-eight-day cycle and are positive of the exact day that sperm met egg, gestational dating can be fuzzy at best. If you are a week or more past the EDD, your provider will order additional tests that will give her a better picture of whether or not baby is ready to arrive.

Babies who stay in the womb forty-two weeks or longer are considered post-date. Postdate pregnancies can develop macrosomia, or large body size (8 pounds, 13 ounces or more) that could make it difficult to pass through the birth canal. A postdate fetus may also pass meconium, which, if released into the amniotic fluid, has the potential to cause lung problems after birth. Postdate pregnancies are also associated with an increased risk of stillbirth and placental insufficiency (when the placenta can no longer provide enough oxygen and nutrients to the baby). That's why regular assessment of a postdate pregnancy is extremely important.

Chapter 15

Labor and Delivery

Even if you've read up on labor and delivery, taken copious notes in every session of childbirth class, and questioned your friends on their birth experiences, you'll still find your labor is different in some way from that of others. Because every woman's labor is unique (as is each birth), comparisons of length, progress, and pain perception can be inaccurate and even discouraging. Follow your own path, and you'll do fine.

Get Ready: Baby and Your Body in Labor

Labor is hard work (don't let anyone tell you otherwise), but it's also some of the most rewarding work you'll ever do.

Contractions

The first signal of labor is contractions—the tightening and releasing of your uterus that helps propel your baby down the birth canal. These contractions differ from the Braxton-Hicks ones you've possibly had in that they occur at regular intervals, are painful, and are slowly but surely opening the door (that is, cervix) for baby's exit.

> If you don't want to be bound to your bed during labor, find out whether your birth facility has fetal monitors that use telemetry. These wireless monitors strap on like a regular external device so that you don't have to remain plugged into anything. There are even telemetry units that are waterproof, so you can use them if you plan on easing labor pains with hydrotherapy.

When contractions start, call your practitioner to let her know labor has started and how far apart contractions are. Remember, contractions are timed from the beginning of one to the start of the next. Your provider will let you know at what point you should head for the hospital or birthing center.

Prep

When you do arrive at your birthing center or hospital, the nursing staff will prep (or prepare) you for labor and delivery. You'll start by changing into your hospital gown or nightgown from home. Depending on your facility's policy, you could be getting a partial shave of your perineal area or, less commonly, a full shave of both your abdominal and pubic area.

Your nurse may insert a needle with a heparin lock and secure it with surgical tape. If intravenous (IV) medication is suddenly needed during labor, it can be easily hooked up. Other hospitals will hook you up to an IV line as a matter of course and administer a glucose solution to keep you hydrated. Other medications can be added to the line as necessary. You may be hooked up to fetal and uterine monitors that will allow you and your coach to see when a contraction is coming and, more importantly, when it seems to be almost over. It will also pick up fetal heart sounds and alert your medical team to any stress the baby may be experiencing. An internal monitor might be used if you are considered to be at high risk.

Get Set: Pain-Relief Options

In early labor when contractions are getting intense but are still not close enough to leave for the hospital, there are a few ways you can ease the pain.

Nonmedical Solutions

Experiment with different positions, such as on all fours, against a wall, and leaning against someone or something while bent forward at the waist.

Back labor, which occurs when baby's face is toward your abdomen rather than toward your spine, can cause severe lower back pain. Ask your partner to try massage or a warm water bottle to ease contractions. The soothing jets of a whirlpool tub, if you have one, can do wonders. If your water has broken, however, never take a soak without approval from your provider.

Keep positive, supportive people around you. Let your coach be your buffer and clear out any distractions. Try to remain focused on riding through and past the contraction. Fix your eyes on something that relaxes you and practice the breathing exercises you learned in childbirth class to keep the oxygen and blood flowing. Don't hyperventilate. Talk or groan through the peak of the contraction if it helps. Letting go in between contractions can help ease your mind and body and loosen you up for impending delivery. Use the relaxation exercises that you learned in childbirth class.

Pharmaceutical Options

Once you arrive at the hospital, you will have analgesics and anesthetics available for pain relief, if you choose to use them.

Analgesics

Analgesics deaden the pain by depressing your nervous system. They make you sleepy and help you rest between contractions. The analgesics Demerol (meperidine), Stadol (butorphanol), Nubain (nalbuphine), and Sublimaze (fentanyl) are commonly used in labor. Although these medications can cross the placenta, when they are properly administered in the appropriate dosages they should not cause baby any serious side effects.

Local Anesthesia

Local anesthesia, also called regional anesthesia, numbs only a specific portion of the body and leaves you awake and alert. The most commonly used local anesthesia is probably the lumbar epidural. Injected into the space between two vertebrae of your lower back (the epidural space), this type of anesthesia is administered when you are well into labor, and it will temporarily numb the nerves all the way from your belly button to your knees. An epidural takes twenty minutes to start working and can lower your blood pressure. For this reason, you'll be put on the fetal monitor and hooked up to an IV fluid drip if you're given an epidural. The numbness will take several hours to wear off and may restrict your movements during the birth, but an epidural can be a great pain-management tool.

A spinal block is similar to an epidural in that it's administered in the lower back. However, a spinal is delivered directly into your lower spine, not into the spaces between your vertebrae as in an epidural. Used right at delivery only or during a cesarean section, the spinal will numb you all the way from your rib cage down.

Women who want the pain-relief benefits of an epidural but also to retain the ability to move around during labor are candidates for a low-dose combination spinal epidural, sometimes referred to as a *walking epidural*. A walking epidural is usually faster acting than a conventional epidural and allows you to retain enough sensation to move and walk, which can speed the labor process.

General Anesthesia

General anesthesia is rarely used in labor and delivery, except in cases of an emergency cesarean section when there isn't adequate time to prep the patient with a local anesthetic. It brings about a complete loss of consciousness. Newborns arriving under the influence of a general anesthesia can be drowsy and slow to respond.

Go! Labor in Three Acts

Labor is a series of three distinct stages, aptly called *first*, *second*, and *third* stages. For most women, the longest span is the first stage, which lasts from the earliest signs of labor right through baby's descent into the birth canal in preparation for stage two—pushing. Stage three consists of delivering the placenta, which mothers usually feel is a cakewalk after all the hard work involved in baby's arrival.

First Stage

The first stage of labor begins with early labor and ends with active labor. Your provider probably uses the term *transition* (or *descent*) to refer to the end of the first stage of labor.

During the early phase the cervix effaces (thins) and dilates (opens). This process may have started several weeks ago. Now your cervix will dilate to 4–5 centimeters. Contractions will arrive every fifteen to twenty minutes and last sixty to ninety seconds. Try to stay up and moving through contractions as much as you can to let gravity help your baby descend. Use the breathing and relaxation techniques you picked up in childbirth class to get you through these first few hours. Then leave for the hospital and the next phase—active labor.

In active labor, your contractions are coming closer together regularly, perhaps three to five minutes apart, and they can be intense, lasting forty-five to sixty seconds. These strong contractions are dilating your cervix from about 4–5 centimeters to around 8.

If your birthing center or hospital has whirlpool tubs or showers available for laboring moms, you might find the pulsating water welcome relief for getting through contractions. This pain-relief method (called *hydrotherapy*) is not the same as a water birth, in which a baby is actually born submerged in a pool of water.

Don't feel inadequate or guilty about asking for pain medication at any point if you want it. Pain medication is a tool, just like your breathing exercises. Wisely used, it can result in a better birth experience for both you and your child.

Once your cervix reaches 8 centimeters and contractions start coming one on top of the other to get you to full dilation, the end of the first stage has arrived. Because of the frequency of contractions and the overwhelming urge to push, this is the most difficult part of labor. Fortunately, it culminates in your child's delivery, once you bridge those final 2 centimeters to become fully dilated.

As you begin to transition from first- to second-stage labor:

- You could be nauseated and may even vomit.
- You have chills or sweats, and your muscles twitch.
- Your back really, really hurts.
- Contractions are just minutes apart, or even less than that.
- There is pressure in your rectum from the baby.
- You are absolutely exhausted.
- You may feel like pushing even though your cervix is not yet fully dilated.

Although every fiber of your body is probably screaming for you to push, you need to hold back just a few moments more. Your cervix is almost but not quite open far enough for baby's safe passage. Take quick, shallow breaths and resist the urge to push until your doctor or midwife gives the go-ahead sign.

Second Stage (or PUSH!)

Your cervix has made it to 10 centimeters, and you are finally allowed to push. This second stage can last anywhere from a few minutes (with second or subsequent babies) to several hours. Your contractions will still arrive regularly, but they aren't quite as close together—a welcome relief. Pushing is very hard work, but the sensations may change from the intense gripping you've experienced to more of a stinging or burning sensation.

> If possible, try to find a pushing position that makes you feel comfortable and in control. Use gravity to your advantage by kneeling, squatting, or sitting up with your legs and knees spread far apart. Stirrups are likely available, but don't feel forced into using them if they don't work for you.

Your birth attendant and/or coach will let you know when the peak of the contraction occurs, the optimum time for pushing effectively. Use whatever it takes to push effectively. If that means moaning, grunting, and emitting other primal sounds that make your prenatal snoring sound like a lullaby by comparison, go for it. The people attending your birth have probably heard just about everything. Don't be embarrassed, because the noise won't even faze them.

You may be asked to stop pushing momentarily as the baby's head is ready to emerge, in order to prevent perineal tearing. Panting can help you suppress the urge. The obstetrician or midwife may decide on an episiotomy if your skin doesn't appear willing to stretch another millimeter, or she may attempt perineal massage.

Finally, the head slides facedown past the perineum and is eased out carefully to prevent injury to the baby. The attendant may wipe the eyes, nose, and mouth and suction any mucus or fluid from her upper respiratory tract. It's all downhill from here as the rest of the body slides out.

As your baby leaves the quiet, dim warmth of the womb, his respiratory reflexes kick in and the newborn lungs fill with air for the first time. He'll probably test out those lungs with a full-fledged wail. Your doctor will place the baby on your stomach for introductions, usually with the umbilical cord still attached.

Third Stage (or You Aren't Done Yet!)

The third stage of labor is the delivery of the placenta. The entire placenta must be expelled to prevent bleeding and infection complications later on. Contractions will continue, and your doctor may press down on your abdomen and massage your uterus or tug gently on the end of the umbilical cord hanging from your vagina. You might also be injected with the hormone Pitocin (oxytocin) to step up your contractions and expel the placenta. Once the placenta is out, any stitches you require to repair tearing or episiotomy incisions will be put in. A local anesthetic will be injected to deaden the area if you aren't still anesthetized from an epidural.

Cesarean Section

A cesarean birth will be scheduled for you if you have a breech baby or other complications or conditions that indicate the need for such. It may also be performed in emergency situations in which the fetus is in distress. A cesarean section (also called a C-section) is major abdominal surgery and carries with it all the risks of infection and complication that any surgical procedure does. On the positive side, with a planned cesarean section, the date your physician schedules the procedure is your due date, and no contractions are necessary unless you begin to labor before that time.

In Advance of the Surgery

If you have any advance warning about your cesarean section, you'll probably be offered an epidural or spinal rather than general anesthesia. Before the procedure begins, you'll be prepped. A nurse may shave the area of the incision, and your arm will be hooked up to an intravenous line to receive fluids as well as pain medication. You may also be asked to drink an antacid solution called *sodium citrate* to neutralize your stomach acid.

Before the procedure begins, you will have a catheter inserted into your bladder. The anesthetic block will give you little control over the muscles that control urine flow, so the catheter will do the work for you both during and after the procedure. Catheter insertion can be uncomfortable, so ask that it be inserted after you've received your anesthetic block (which will likely be in the operating room).

In the Operating Room

Once you're prepped, you will be wheeled to the operating room. In the operating room, the anesthesiologist will place the epidural or spinal block into your back. You'll then be asked to lie flat on your back with your arms straight out to the sides. A curtain just a few feet high will be positioned at your chest to keep the surgical field (the area where all the action is) sterile. This will also block your view of the procedure, so if you're determined to see baby the moment she emerges, you will want to ask for an appropriately placed mirror as early as possible.

Your arms may be loosely fastened down with Velcro straps. This is to prevent any accidental movements that could breach the sterility of the surgical field.

The most uncomfortable part of the cesarean section procedure is arguably the flat-on-your-back part. It's quite possible you will get nauseated as your heavy uterus compresses your vena cava and starts to lower your blood pressure. In addition, the anesthetic itself may cause your blood pressure to fall. Although the anesthesiologist will administer medication to control this drop (called *hypotension*), you may get sick to your stomach. The discomfort is compounded by the fact that you will have to vomit lying down with your head turned to the side. This is where a well-placed mate, tray in hand, is indispensable. Hang in there and remember this part will likely be short lived.

The obstetrician will make an incision, and the baby's head, perfectly round because she hasn't done battle with the birth canal, will be lifted out first and her mouth and nose suctioned. As your doctor helps your baby out of the incision, you'll feel a strange pulling sensation. Once the cord is cut, you'll be able to finally see your baby, albeit briefly, before he is taken for assessment and a quick cleanup by the nursing staff. In some cases the pediatric team will be in the operating room to assess the baby immediately. Your incision will be stitched closed, and you'll be wheeled off to the recovery room where your little one will meet up with you once again. The entire surgical procedure will take only about thirty to forty-five minutes.

Emergency Cesarean Section

If your cesarean section is performed under emergency circumstances, events could move quickly and you'll have fewer options. You could also be given a general anesthetic that will make you unconscious. Most partners are asked to step outside once general anesthesia has been administered, but you might want to talk to your doctor about special circumstances during childbirth.

Induction

In cases where you are definitely forty-one weeks or farther along and it seems your child is perfectly content to spend his infancy in your womb, your practitioner may recommend induction. Inducing labor involves both helping the cervix ripen for baby's passage and stimulating uterine contractions; both are important for a successful labor and delivery.

Your provider may use one of several methods to facilitate cervical ripening, including membrane stripping and amniotomy (manual breaking of the membranes or bag of waters). Stripping (or sweeping) of the membranes is simply the separation of the amniotic membrane from the wall of the cervix. Your provider will insert her finger in the cervix and gently sweep it between the amniotic membrane and the uterine wall.

If she opts for amniotomy, she'll use an instrument with a small blunt hook on the end to break through the amniotic sac. With the latter method, if labor does not start on its own within twenty-four hours, scheduled induction may be necessary because of the risk of infection for the baby.

Because a scheduled induction is more successful when the cervix is prepared for the experience, your practitioner may recommend an application of prostaglandin to your cervix the day prior or in the hospital. The prostaglandin helps ripen the cervix for labor and delivery. In some cases it can be used alone as an inducing agent. The prostaglandin can take the form of a gel or tablet and can be inserted into the vagina. On some occasions, the tablet is given orally. The baby's heart rate is assessed with a fetal monitor after the prostaglandin is given and during labor. More than one application may be ordered.

Manual dilators and Foley catheters can also be used for cervical ripening as an alternative to the use of drugs. The type of cervical ripening method used depends on your personal preference, your medical history, and the cervical exam.

Pitocin, a synthetic formulation of the hormone oxytocin that stimulates uterine contractions, may be prescribed as an inducing agent. The hormone is given intravenously, and you will be hooked up to a fetal monitor to monitor your baby's progress.

According to the CDC, more than one in five births were induced in 2005. Researchers attribute the increase to earlier prenatal care, wider availability of induction agents, and nonmedical reasons such as convenience for the patient or doctor. Because induction can cause intense contractions and result in a longer labor, its use should always be carefully considered.

After the Birth

The pinnacle of nine months of physical chaos and emotional oscillation, queasy stomach, aches, pains, and hair-trigger laughter and tears has arrived. Your baby is here, placed skin-to-skin to feel his mother's outside warmth for the very first time.

Meeting Baby

A thousand different feelings and emotions, from utter exhaustion to indescribable joy, will flood you as you look down at that little scrunched face, still adjusting to his new waterless environment. Wrapped in a blanket with a little stocking cap to keep his head warm, he looks so perfect yet so vulnerable.

If you're planning on breastfeeding, you can nurse him while you get acquainted, even in the recovery room if you've had a cesarean section. It's awe inspiring how he knows just what to do, instinctively rooting for your breast with his eyes barely open and then latching on. Spend as long as you want getting familiar, and let your partner share in the bonding too. This is a precious time for your new family.

Baby's First Doctor's Visit

Your baby will have some initial tests and treatments to ensure a healthy welcome into the world. The first is an Apgar test. Created by noted pediatrician Dr. Virginia Apgar, this test measures appearance (skin color), pulse, grimace (reflexes), activity, and respiration. It is given just one minute after birth and again five minutes after that. The attendant will assign a score of 0 to 2 for each category and add the numbers together for the total Apgar score; average scores are 7–10.

After the Apgar test, your newborn will be measured, weighed, and have prints taken of her feet and fingers. Silver nitrate or antibiotic eye drops or ointment may be put in her eyes to prevent infection from anything she encountered in the birth canal. She'll also receive a vitamin K injection to prevent bleeding problems, a heel-stick blood draw to test for PKU and hypothyroidism, and in some hospitals a hepatitis B vaccine. Further tests may be administered if you have a chronic illness or have experienced complications during pregnancy.

Taking Care of Mom

After the birth, you'll have some assistance cleaning up and will be given a good supply of superabsorbent sanitary pads. You'll also be provided with a perineal irrigation bottle, a plastic squirt bottle used to cleanse and soothe your perineal area with warm water each time you use the bathroom.

If bleeding is soaking more than a pad an hour, let your provider know. It could be a sign that a piece of placenta is still retained in your uterus. This condition usually requires surgical removal of the placental fragments, called *curettage*.

You'll be expelling lochia for up to six weeks following birth, whether you've had a vaginal birth or a cesarean section. Lochia—a mixture of blood, mucus, and tissue that comes from the implantation site of the placenta—will be quite heavy in the days immediately following the birth, so don't be alarmed.

If you've had a cesarean section, you'll spend some time in the recovery area before heading to your hospital room. Your incision will be checked regularly and pain medication will be administered as needed. The next day you'll be encouraged to walk as soon as possible to get your digestive tract active again, and you'll be asked about your gas and bathroom habits ad nauseam. The nursing staff is just trying to ensure that everything is returning to normal in gastrointestinal land.

Women who are given episiotomies will take sitz baths (also known as *hip baths*) to relieve pain, promote healing, and keep the area clean. A sitz bath is a small shallow tub of water, sometimes with medication added, that you sit in. Some mild pain relievers may also be prescribed to ease episiotomy pain.

If you are planning on breastfeeding, now is the perfect time to get your technique down. Your OB nurses will likely ask you how breastfeeding is progressing and can examine your latching technique to help you troubleshoot if breastfeeding isn't yet going smoothly. In some cases, there is even a lactation consultant available, and hospitals frequently offer breastfeeding classes to their new-mother inpatients.

Remember that even though it will take a few days for your breasts to start manufacturing milk, you are still providing your child with nutrient-rich colostrum, the prelude to breast milk. When your milk does come in, about the third day after delivery, your breasts can be quite swollen, hard, and sore. This engorgement will be relieved upon nursing. If you're going the bottle route, cold packs and supportive bras or binding can ease the discomfort. The tenderness of engorgement usually passes in two to three days and can be relieved by mild analgesics as prescribed by your doctor.

Conclusion

Now you have a new baby to care for! Your hard work and vegan diet during pregnancy has paid off. Whether you are a new mom or have other children, this time can be overwhelming. Eating properly can be challenging but is essential for your own health and the health of your child. The following section of the book contains easy vegan recipes to follow. Enjoy!

Part 5

Recipes

Chapter 16

Vegan Breakfasts

Quick Tofu Breakfast Burrito

INGREDIENTS

Serves 4

1 (16-ounce) block extra-firm tofu, well pressed

2 tablespoons olive oil

½ cup mild salsa

½ teaspoon chili powder

⅛ teaspoon salt

⅛ teaspoon black pepper

4 (6") vegan flour tortillas, warmed

4 slices vegan Cheddar cheese

1 medium avocado, peeled, pitted, and sliced

1. Cube or crumble tofu into 1" chunks. Sauté chunks in olive oil in a medium skillet over medium heat for 2–3 minutes.
2. Add salsa and chili powder and cook for 2–3 more minutes, stirring frequently. Season with salt and pepper.
3. Layer each warmed tortilla with ¼ tofu mixture.
4. Add vegan cheese and avocado slices and wrap like a burrito.

Per Serving
Calories: 362 | Fat: 21.1 grams | Sodium: 686 milligrams
Fiber: 4.1 grams | Carbohydrates: 28.8 grams
Net Carbohydrates: 24.7 grams | Sugar: 3.7 grams
Protein: 15.3 grams

ADD SOME SAUCE
Adding ketchup or hot sauce is a great way to spice this recipe up. Before you wrap up your burrito, drizzle a teaspoon or more of ketchup or hot sauce over the tofu. Yum!

Maple Cinnamon Breakfast Quinoa

INGREDIENTS

Serves 4

1 cup dry quinoa, rinsed and drained

2 cups water

1 teaspoon vegan margarine

⅔ cup unsweetened soy milk

½ teaspoon ground cinnamon

2 tablespoons maple syrup

2 tablespoons raisins

2 large bananas, peeled and sliced

1. In a small saucepan, bring quinoa and water to a boil over high heat. Reduce to a simmer and allow to cook covered for 15 minutes until liquid is absorbed.
2. Remove from heat and fluff quinoa with a fork. Cover and allow to sit for 5 minutes.
3. Stir in margarine and soy milk, then remaining ingredients.

Per Serving
Calories: 276 | Fat: 3.6 grams | Sodium: 25 milligrams
Fiber: 5.3 grams | Carbohydrates: 54.6 grams
Net Carbohydrates: 49.3 grams | Sugar: 17.6 grams
Protein: 8.1 grams

Vegan Pancakes

INGREDIENTS

Yields 1 Dozen Pancakes

1 cup all-purpose flour
1 tablespoon sugar
1¾ teaspoons baking powder
¼ teaspoon salt
½ large banana, peeled
1 teaspoon vanilla extract
1 cup unsweetened soy milk

1. In a large bowl, mix together flour, sugar, baking powder, and salt.
2. In a small bowl, mash banana with a fork. Add vanilla; whisk until smooth and fluffy. Add soy milk; stir to combine well.
3. Add wet mixture to dry ingredients, then stir.
4. Grease a griddle or large frying pan with vegetable cooking spray and heat over medium heat. Drop batter about 3 tablespoons at a time and heat until bubbles appear on surface, about 2–3 minutes. Flip and cook other side until lightly golden brown, another 1–2 minutes.

Per Pancake
Calories: 54 | Fat: 0.4 grams | Sodium: 127 milligrams
Fiber: 0.5 grams | Carbohydrates: 10.9 grams
Net Carbohydrates: 10.4 grams | Sugar: 1.9 grams
Protein: 1.7 grams

Apple Cinnamon Waffles

INGREDIENTS

Serves 4

1¼ cups all-purpose flour
2 teaspoons baking powder
½ teaspoon ground cinnamon
2 teaspoons sugar
1 cup unsweetened soy milk
½ cup unsweetened
    applesauce
1 teaspoon vanilla extract
1 tablespoon vegetable oil

1. In a large bowl, combine flour, baking powder, cinnamon, and sugar. Set aside.
2. In a small bowl, combine soy milk, applesauce, vanilla, and oil.
3. Add soy milk mixture to dry ingredients, stirring just until combined; do not overmix.
4. Carefully drop about ¼ cup batter onto preheated waffle iron for each waffle and cook until done, about 5–7 minutes.

Per Serving
Calories: 218 | Fat: 4.5 grams | Sodium: 267 milligrams
Fiber: 1.9 grams | Carbohydrates: 37.4 grams
Net Carbohydrates: 35.5 grams | Sugar: 5.5 grams
Protein: 5.8 grams

Super Green Quiche

INGREDIENTS

Serves 4

1 (10-ounce) package frozen chopped spinach, thawed and drained

½ cup diced broccoli

1 (16-ounce) block firm or extra-firm tofu

1 tablespoon soy sauce

¼ cup unsweetened soy milk

1 teaspoon prepared mustard

2 tablespoons nutritional yeast

½ teaspoon garlic powder

1 teaspoon dried parsley

½ teaspoon dried rosemary

¾ teaspoon salt

¼ teaspoon black pepper

1 store-bought vegan pie crust

1. Preheat oven to 350°F.
2. Steam spinach and broccoli approximately 4 minutes until just lightly cooked, then set aside to cool. Press as much moisture as possible out of spinach.
3. In a blender or food processor, combine tofu with remaining ingredients except crust until well mixed. Mix in spinach and broccoli by hand until combined.
4. Spread mixture evenly in pie crust.
5. Bake for 35–40 minutes until firm. Allow to cool for at least 10 minutes before serving. Quiche will firm up a bit more as it cools.

Per Serving
Calories: 385 | Fat: 21.1 grams | Sodium: 932 milligrams
Fiber: 4.1 grams | Carbohydrates: 35.5 grams
Net Carbohydrates: 31.4 grams | Sugar: 5.5 grams
Protein: 16.5 grams

Whole-Wheat Blueberry Muffins

INGREDIENTS

Yields about 1½ Dozen Muffins

2 cups whole-wheat flour
1 cup all-purpose flour
1¼ cups sugar
1 tablespoon baking powder
1 teaspoon salt
1½ cups unsweetened soy milk
½ cup unsweetened applesauce
½ teaspoon vanilla extract
2 cups blueberries, divided

1. Preheat oven to 400°F.
2. In a large bowl, combine flours, sugar, baking powder, and salt. Set aside.
3. In a small bowl, whisk together soy milk, applesauce, and vanilla until well mixed.
4. Combine wet ingredients with dry ingredients; stir just until mixed. Gently fold in ½ of the blueberries.
5. Spoon batter into lined muffin tins, filling each muffin compartment about ⅔ full. Sprinkle remaining blueberries on top of muffins.
6. Bake for 20–25 minutes until lightly golden brown on top.

Per Muffin
Calories: 143 | Fat: 0.7 grams | Sodium: 218 milligrams
Fiber: 2.2 grams | Carbohydrates: 32.5 grams
Net Carbohydrates: 30.3 grams | Sugar: 16.3 grams
Protein: 3.2 grams

....

MAKING VEGAN MUFFINS

Got a favorite muffin recipe? Try making it vegan! Use a commercial egg replacer in place of the eggs and substitute a vegan soy margarine and soy milk for the butter and milk. Voilà!

....

Chapter 17

Entrées

Barley Baked Beans

INGREDIENTS

Serves 8

2 cups cooked barley

2 (15-ounce) cans navy beans, drained and rinsed

1 medium yellow onion, peeled and diced

1 (28-ounce) can crushed tomatoes

½ cup water

¼ cup dark brown sugar

⅓ cup barbecue sauce

2 tablespoons molasses

2 teaspoons mustard powder

1 teaspoon garlic powder

1 teaspoon salt

1. Preheat oven to 300°F.
2. In a large (10-cup or larger) casserole or baking dish sprayed with vegetable cooking spray, combine all ingredients. Cover and bake for 2 hours, stirring occasionally.
3. Uncover and bake for about 15 more minutes until thick and saucy.

Per Serving
Calories: 281 | Fat: 1.0 grams | Sodium: 905 milligrams
Fiber: 9.6 grams | Carbohydrates: 59.0 grams
Net Carbohydrates: 49.4 grams | Sugar: 20.1 grams
Protein: 11.6 grams

Chickpea Soft Tacos

INGREDIENTS

Serves 4

2 (15-ounce) cans chickpeas, drained and rinsed
½ cup water
1 (6-ounce) can tomato paste
1 tablespoon chili powder
1 teaspoon garlic powder
½ teaspoon onion powder
½ teaspoon cumin
¼ cup chopped fresh cilantro
4 (6") vegan flour tortillas

1. In a large skillet, combine chickpeas, water, tomato paste, chili powder, garlic powder, onion powder, and cumin. Cover and simmer over medium heat for 10 minutes, stirring occasionally. Uncover and simmer 1–2 minutes until most of the liquid is absorbed.
2. Use a fork or potato masher to mash chickpeas until half mashed. Stir in cilantro.
3. Spoon mixture into flour tortillas and wrap.

Per Serving
Calories: 315 | Fat: 4.3 grams | Sodium: 577 milligrams
Fiber: 11.7 grams | Carbohydrates: 55.8 grams
Net Carbohydrates: 44.1 grams | Sugar: 11.7 grams
Protein: 14.1 grams

A WORD ABOUT CILANTRO
Not a cilantro fan? That's okay! This recipe will taste great without it. Just omit and enjoy!

Mexico City Protein Bowl

INGREDIENTS

Serves 2

½ block (8 ounces) firm tofu, diced small

1 scallion, chopped

1 tablespoon olive oil

½ cup frozen peas, thawed

½ cup frozen corn kernels, thawed

½ teaspoon chili powder

1 (15-ounce) can black beans, drained and rinsed

2 (6") corn tortillas

1. In a medium skillet over medium-high heat, sauté tofu and scallion in olive oil for 2–3 minutes; add peas, corn, and chili powder. Cook another 1–2 minutes, stirring frequently.
2. Reduce heat to medium-low; add black beans. Cook for 4–5 minutes until well combined and heated through.
3. Place a corn tortilla in the bottom of a bowl; spoon ½ tofu mixture over the top of each.

Per Serving
Calories: 443 | Fat: 12.7 grams | Sodium: 524 milligrams
Fiber: 19.9 grams | Carbohydrates: 59.9 grams
Net Carbohydrates: 40.0 grams | Sugar: 5.8 grams
Protein: 26.6 grams

HOT SAUCE HINT

Craving some heat? Add a splash, no more than a teaspoon, of hot sauce to your protein bowl to kick up the spiciness.

Pasta and Peas

INGREDIENTS

Serves 6

1½ cups unsweetened soy milk
1 teaspoon garlic powder
2 tablespoons vegan
   margarine
1 tablespoon all-purpose flour
1½ cups frozen green peas,
   thawed
⅓ cup nutritional yeast
1 (12-ounce) package whole-
   wheat rotini pasta, cooked
¼ teaspoon salt
⅛ teaspoon black pepper

1. In a medium pot, whisk together soy milk, garlic powder, and margarine over low heat until margarine is melted. Add flour; stir well to combine, heating just until thickened, about 5 minutes.
2. Add peas and nutritional yeast until heated and well mixed, about 5 minutes; pour over pasta.
3. Season with salt and pepper.

Per Serving
Calories: 291 | Fat: 3.3 grams | Sodium: 191 milligrams
Fiber: 4.4 grams | Carbohydrates: 50.6 grams
Net Carbohydrates: 46.2 grams | Sugar: 3.5 grams
Protein: 12.9 grams

Creamy Sun-Dried Tomato Pasta

INGREDIENTS

Serves 6

1 (12-ounce) block silken firm
   tofu, drained
¼ cup unsweetened soy milk
2 tablespoons red wine vinegar
½ teaspoon garlic powder
½ teaspoon salt
1¼ cups sun-dried tomatoes,
   rehydrated
1 teaspoon dried parsley
1 (12-ounce) package
   spaghetti, cooked
2 tablespoons chopped fresh
   basil

1. In a blender or food processor, blend together tofu, soy milk, vinegar, garlic powder, and salt until smooth and creamy, about 1 minute. Add tomatoes and parsley; pulse until tomatoes are finely diced.
2. Transfer sauce to a small pot and heat over medium-low heat just until hot, about 5–10 minutes.
3. Pour sauce over pasta and sprinkle with basil.

Per Serving
Calories: 279 | Fat: 2.3 grams | Sodium: 249 milligrams
Fiber: 3.4 grams | Carbohydrates: 50.4 grams
Net Carbohydrates: 47.0 grams | Sugar: 6.5 grams
Protein: 13.3 grams

Lemon Basil Tofu

INGREDIENTS

Serves 6

3 tablespoons lemon juice
1 tablespoon soy sauce
2 teaspoons apple cider vinegar
1 tablespoon Dijon mustard
¾ teaspoon sugar
3 tablespoons olive oil
2 tablespoons chopped fresh basil, plus extra for garnish, divided
2 (16-ounce) blocks firm or extra-firm tofu, well pressed

1. Whisk together all ingredients except tofu; transfer to an ungreased 9" × 13" baking dish.
2. Slice tofu into ½"-thick strips or triangles.
3. Place tofu in marinade and coat well. Allow to marinate in the refrigerator for at least 1 hour or overnight, being sure tofu is well coated in marinade.
4. Preheat oven to 350°F.
5. Bake for 15 minutes, turn tofu pieces over, then bake for another 12 minutes until most of the marinade is absorbed. Garnish with a few extra bits of chopped fresh basil.

Per Serving
Calories: 176 | Fat: 12.7 grams | Sodium: 227 milligrams
Fiber: 1.4 grams | Carbohydrates: 4.0 grams
Net Carbohydrates: 2.6 grams | Sugar: 1.7 grams
Protein: 12.9 grams

Easy Falafel Patties

INGREDIENTS

Serves 4

1 (15-ounce) can chickpeas, drained and rinsed
½ medium yellow onion, peeled and minced
1 tablespoon all-purpose flour
1 teaspoon cumin
¾ teaspoon garlic powder
¾ teaspoon salt
Egg replacer for 1 egg
¼ cup chopped fresh parsley
2 tablespoons chopped fresh cilantro

1. Preheat oven to 375°F.
2. Place chickpeas in a large bowl and mash with a fork until coarsely mashed, or pulse in a food processor until chopped.
3. Combine chickpeas with onions, flour, cumin, garlic powder, salt, and egg substitute; mash together to combine. Add parsley and cilantro.
4. Shape mixture into eight (1"-thick) patties and place on baking sheet lightly oiled with vegetable cooking spray and bake in oven for about 15 minutes until crisp.

Per Serving (2 Patties)
Calories: 116 | Fat: 1.5 grams | Sodium: 585 milligrams
Fiber: 5.0 grams | Carbohydrates: 19.4 grams
Net Carbohydrates: 14.4 grams | Sugar: 3.6 grams
Protein: 6.1 grams

Balsamic Dijon Orzo

INGREDIENTS

Serves 4

3 tablespoons balsamic vinegar
1½ tablespoons Dijon mustard
1½ tablespoons olive oil
1 teaspoon dried basil
1 teaspoon dried parsley
½ teaspoon dried oregano
1½ cups dry orzo
2 medium red ripe tomatoes,
    cored and chopped
½ cup sliced black olives
1 (15-ounce) can cannellini
    beans, drained and rinsed
½ teaspoon salt
¼ teaspoon black pepper

1. In a small bowl or container, whisk together vinegar, mustard, olive oil, basil, parsley, and oregano until well mixed.
2. Cook orzo according to package instructions.
3. In a medium pot over low heat, combine orzo with balsamic dressing; add tomatoes, olives, and beans. Cook for 3–4 minutes, stirring to combine.
4. Season with salt and pepper.

Per Serving
Calories: 453 | Fat: 8.8 grams | Sodium: 810 milligrams
Fiber: 9.3 grams | Carbohydrates: 77.6 grams
Net Carbohydrates: 68.3 grams | Sugar: 7.3 grams
Protein: 17.6 grams

Tandoori Seitan

INGREDIENTS

Serves 6

⅔ cup plain soy yogurt

2 tablespoons lemon juice

1½ tablespoons tandoori
spice blend

½ teaspoon cumin

½ teaspoon garlic powder

¼ teaspoon salt

1 (16-ounce) package
prepared seitan, chopped
into ¾" pieces

1 medium red bell pepper,
seeded and chopped

1 medium yellow onion,
peeled and chopped

1 medium red ripe tomato,
cored and chopped

2 tablespoons olive oil

1. In a shallow 4-cup bowl or pan, whisk together yogurt, lemon juice, and all spices; add seitan. Allow to marinate in refrigerator for at least 1 hour. Reserve marinade.
2. In a medium skillet over medium-high heat, sauté pepper, onions, and tomato in oil until just barely soft, about 4 minutes.
3. Reduce heat to low; add seitan. Cook, tossing seitan occasionally, for 8–10 minutes.
4. Serve topped with extra marinade.

Per Serving
Calories: 161 | Fat: 4.9 grams | Sodium: 574 milligrams
Fiber: 2.7 grams | Carbohydrates: 14.1 grams
Net Carbohydrates: 11.4 grams | Sugar: 4.5 grams
Protein: 15.2 grams

Tofu "Chicken" Nuggets

INGREDIENTS

Serves 4

¼ cup unsweetened soy milk

2 tablespoons prepared
    mustard

3 tablespoons nutritional yeast

½ cup bread crumbs

½ cup all-purpose flour

1 teaspoon poultry seasoning

1 teaspoon garlic powder

1 teaspoon onion powder

½ teaspoon salt

¼ teaspoon black pepper

1 (16-ounce) block firm or
    extra-firm tofu, sliced into
    thin strips

1. Preheat oven to 375°F.
2. In an 8" shallow square pan, whisk together soy milk, mustard, and nutritional yeast.
3. In a separate medium bowl, combine bread crumbs, flour, poultry seasoning, garlic powder, onion powder, salt, and pepper.
4. Coat each piece of tofu with soy milk mixture, then coat well in bread crumb mixture.
5. Bake for 20 minutes, turning once.

Per Serving
Calories: 157 | Fat: 5.3 grams | Sodium: 303 milligrams
Fiber: 2.6 grams | Carbohydrates: 15.1 grams
Net Carbohydrates: 12.5 grams | Sugar: 1.3 grams
Protein: 13.3 grams

The Easiest Black Bean Burger Recipe in the World

INGREDIENTS

Yields 6 Patties

1 (15-ounce) can black beans, drained and rinsed
3 tablespoons minced peeled onion
1 teaspoon salt
1½ teaspoons garlic powder
2 teaspoons dried parsley
1 teaspoon chili powder
⅔ cup all-purpose flour
2 tablespoons olive oil

1. In a blender or food processor, process beans until halfway mashed (about 10 seconds), or mash with a fork.
2. Remove to a medium bowl and add onions, salt, garlic powder, parsley, and chili powder and mash to combine.
3. Add flour, a bit at a time, again mashing together to combine. You may need a little bit more or less than ⅔ cup. Beans should stick together completely.
4. Form into patties. In a large skillet over medium-high heat, panfry in oil for 2–3 minutes on each side. Patties will appear to be done on the outside while still a bit mushy on the inside, so fry them a few minutes longer than you think they need.

Per Patty
Calories: 159 | Fat: 4.7 grams | Sodium: 559 milligrams
Fiber: 5.5 grams | Carbohydrates: 23.5 grams
Net Carbohydrates: 18.0 grams | Sugar: 0.5 grams
Protein: 5.9 grams

Lentil and Rice Loaf

INGREDIENTS

Serves 6

3 cloves garlic, minced
1 large yellow onion, peeled and diced
2 tablespoons olive oil
3½ cups cooked brown lentils
2¼ cups cooked medium-grain white rice
⅓ cup plus 3 tablespoons ketchup
2 tablespoons all-purpose flour
Egg replacer for 1 egg
½ teaspoon dried parsley
½ teaspoon dried thyme
½ teaspoon dried oregano
¼ teaspoon dried sage
¾ teaspoon salt
½ teaspoon black pepper

1. Preheat oven to 350°F.
2. Sauté garlic and onions in oil in a medium pan over medium-high heat until onions are soft and clear, about 3–4 minutes.
3. In a large bowl, use a fork or potato masher to mash lentils until about ⅔ mashed.
4. Add garlic and onions, rice, ⅓ cup ketchup, and flour; combine well. Add egg replacer and seasonings; mash to combine.
5. Gently press mixture into a 9" × 5" × 3" loaf pan lightly greased with vegetable cooking spray. Drizzle remaining 3 tablespoons ketchup on top.
6. Bake for 60 minutes. Allow to cool at least 10 minutes before serving, as loaf will firm slightly as it cools.

Per Serving
Calories: 313 | Fat: 5.0 grams | Sodium: 495 milligrams
Fiber: 10.2 grams | Carbohydrates: 54.5 grams
Net Carbohydrates: 44.3 grams | Sugar: 8.0 grams
Protein: 13.5 grams

Easy Pad Thai Noodles

INGREDIENTS

Serves 4

1 pound thin rice noodles
¼ cup tahini
¼ cup ketchup
¼ cup soy sauce
2 tablespoons rice vinegar
3 tablespoons lime juice
2 tablespoons sugar
¾ teaspoon crushed red
  pepper flakes
1 (16-ounce) block firm or
  extra-firm tofu, diced small
3 cloves garlic, minced
¼ cup vegetable oil
4 scallions, chopped
½ teaspoon salt

1. Cover noodles in hot water and set aside to soak until soft, about 5 minutes.
2. In a small bowl, whisk together tahini, ketchup, soy sauce, vinegar, lime juice, sugar, and red pepper flakes.
3. In a large skillet over medium-high heat, sauté tofu and garlic in oil until tofu is lightly golden brown, about 8–10 minutes. Add drained noodles, stirring to combine well; cook for 2–3 minutes.
4. Reduce heat to medium; add tahini mixture, stirring well to combine. Allow to cook for 3–4 minutes until well combined and heated through. Add scallions and salt and heat 1 more minute, stirring well.

Per Serving
Calories: 692 | Fat: 18.4 grams | Sodium: 1,533 milligrams
Fiber: 4.6 grams | Carbohydrates: 109.6 grams
Net Carbohydrates: 105.0 grams | Sugar: 10.7 grams
Protein: 20.3 grams

ADD SOME TOPPINGS
Optional toppings for this recipe include extra scallions, crushed toasted peanuts, and sliced lime.

Sesame Baked Tofu

INGREDIENTS

Serves 6

¼ cup soy sauce

2 tablespoons sesame oil

¾ teaspoon garlic powder

½ teaspoon ginger powder

2 (16-ounce) blocks firm or extra-firm tofu, well pressed

1. In a small bowl, whisk together soy sauce, sesame oil, garlic powder, and ginger powder; transfer to a wide, shallow 9" × 14" pan.
2. Slice tofu into ½"-thick strips or triangles.
3. Place tofu in marinade and coat well. Allow to marinate in refrigerator for at least 1 hour or overnight.
4. Preheat oven to 400°F.
5. Coat a baking sheet well with vegetable cooking spray or olive oil, or line with foil. Place tofu on sheet.
6. Bake for 20–25 minutes; turn over and bake for another 10–15 minutes until most of marinade is absorbed.

Per Serving
Calories: 110 | Fat: 6.3 grams | Sodium: 76 milligrams
Fiber: 1.4 grams | Carbohydrates: 2.6 grams
Net Carbohydrates: 1.2 grams | Sugar: 0.9 grams
Protein: 12.5 grams

MARINATING TOFU
For marinated baked tofu dishes, a zip-top bag can be helpful in getting the tofu well covered with marinade. Place the tofu in the bag, pour the marinade in, seal, and set in the refrigerator, occasionally turning and lightly shaking to coat all sides of the tofu.

Chapter 18

Sides: Grains

Coconut Rice

INGREDIENTS

Serves 4

1 cup water
1 (14-ounce) can coconut milk
1½ cups white rice, uncooked
⅓ cup unsweetened coconut flakes
1 teaspoon lime juice
½ teaspoon salt

1. In a large pot, combine water, coconut milk, and rice; bring to a simmer over high heat. Reduce heat to medium-low, cover, and allow to cook about 20 minutes until rice reaches desired doneness.
2. In a small skillet, toast coconut flakes over low heat until lightly golden, about 3 minutes. Gently stir constantly to avoid burning.
3. Combine coconut flakes with cooked rice; stir in lime juice and salt.

Per Serving
Calories: 507 | Fat: 24.7 grams | Sodium: 305 milligrams
Fiber: 0.9 grams | Carbohydrates: 62.7 grams
Net Carbohydrates: 61.8 grams | Sugar: 0.2 grams
Protein: 7.3 grams

Baked Millet Patties

INGREDIENTS

Yields 8 Patties

1½ cups cooked millet
½ cup tahini
1 cup bread crumbs
1 teaspoon dried parsley
¾ teaspoon garlic powder
½ teaspoon onion powder
⅓ teaspoon salt

1. Preheat oven to 350°F.
2. Combine all ingredients together in a large bowl; mash to mix well.
3. Use your hands to press firmly into patties, about 1" thick. Place on a baking sheet greased with vegetable cooking spray.
4. Bake for 10–12 minutes on each side.

Per Patty
Calories: 178 | Fat: 7.7 grams | Sodium: 207 milligrams
Fiber: 2.5 grams | Carbohydrates: 21.7 grams
Net Carbohydrates: 19.2 grams | Sugar: 0.9 grams
Protein: 5.7 grams

Lemon Cilantro Couscous

INGREDIENTS

Serves 4

2 cups vegetable broth
1 cup couscous
⅓ cup lemon juice
½ cup chopped fresh cilantro
¼ teaspoon salt

1. In a medium pot over high heat, bring broth to a simmer; add couscous. Turn off heat, cover, and let stand for 10 minutes until soft. Fluff with a fork.
2. Stir in lemon juice, cilantro, and salt.

Per Serving
Calories: 176 | Fat: 0.2 grams | Sodium: 420 milligrams
Fiber: 2.8 grams | Carbohydrates: 37.2 grams
Net Carbohydrates: 34.4 grams | Sugar: 1.3 grams
Protein: 5.7 grams

Mexican Rice with Corn and Peppers

INGREDIENTS

Serves 4

2 cloves garlic, minced
1 cup white rice, uncooked
2 tablespoons olive oil
2 cups vegetable broth
1 cup tomato paste
1 medium green bell pepper, seeded and chopped
1 medium red bell pepper, seeded and chopped
Kernels from 1 medium ear of corn
1 medium carrot, peeled and diced
1 teaspoon chili powder
½ teaspoon cumin
⅓ teaspoon dried oregano
⅓ teaspoon cayenne pepper
⅓ teaspoon salt

1. In a large skillet over medium-high heat, add garlic, rice, and olive oil. Toast rice, stirring frequently until just golden brown, about 2–3 minutes.
2. Reduce heat to medium and add remaining ingredients.
3. Bring to a simmer, cover, and allow to cook until liquid is absorbed and rice is cooked, about 20–25 minutes, stirring occasionally.

Per Serving
Calories: 344 | Fat: 7.6 grams | Sodium: 538 milligrams
Fiber: 5.6 grams | Carbohydrates: 63.2 grams
Net Carbohydrates: 57.6 grams | Sugar: 12.9 grams
Protein: 7.9 grams

VEGAN BURRITOS
Brown some vegetarian chorizo or mock sausage crumbles, mix with Mexican Rice with Corn and Peppers, and wrap in tortillas, perhaps topped with some shredded vegan cheese, to make vegan burritos.

Mediterranean Quinoa Pilaf

INGREDIENTS

Serves 4

1½ cups quinoa, rinsed and drained
3 cups vegetable broth
3 tablespoons balsamic vinegar
2 tablespoons olive oil
1 tablespoon lemon juice
⅓ teaspoon salt
½ cup chopped sun-dried tomatoes
½ cup chopped canned artichoke hearts
½ cup sliced black olives

1. In a large saucepan, bring quinoa and broth to a boil over high heat; reduce to a simmer. Cover and allow quinoa to cook until liquid is absorbed, about 15 minutes. Remove from heat, fluff quinoa with a fork, and allow to stand another 5 minutes.
2. Stir in vinegar, olive oil, lemon juice, and salt; add remaining ingredients, gently tossing to combine.

Per Serving
Calories: 374 | Fat: 13.3 grams | Sodium: 815 milligrams
Fiber: 7.3 grams | Carbohydrates: 53.1 grams
Net Carbohydrates: 45.8 grams | Sugar: 5.4 grams
Protein: 10.8 grams

Millet and Butternut Squash Casserole

INGREDIENTS

Serves 4

1 cup millet
2 cups vegetable broth
1 small butternut squash, peeled, seeded, and chopped
½ cup water
1 teaspoon curry powder
½ cup orange juice
2 tablespoons nutritional yeast
½ teaspoon sea salt

1. Combine millet and broth in a small pot. Bring to a boil over high heat. Cover, decrease heat to low and simmer until done, about 20 minutes.
2. In a medium pan over medium-high heat, heat butternut squash in water. Cover and allow to cook for 10–15 minutes, until squash is almost soft. Remove lid and drain extra water.
3. Combine millet with squash over low heat; add curry powder and orange juice, stirring to combine well.
4. Heat for 3–4 more minutes; add nutritional yeast and salt.

Per Serving
Calories: 282 | Fat: 2.1 grams | Sodium: 476 milligrams
Fiber: 8.3 grams | Carbohydrates: 58.4 grams
Net Carbohydrates: 40.1 grams | Sugar: 6.2 grams
Protein: 8.2 grams

"Cheesy" Broccoli and Rice Casserole

INGREDIENTS

Serves 4

1 head broccoli, chopped small

1 medium yellow onion, peeled and chopped

4 cloves garlic, minced

2 tablespoons olive oil

2 tablespoons all-purpose flour

2 cups unsweetened soy milk

½ cup vegetable broth

2 tablespoons nutritional yeast

1 tablespoon vegan margarine

¼ teaspoon ground nutmeg

¼ teaspoon mustard powder

½ teaspoon salt

3½ cups cooked medium-grain white rice

⅔ cup bread crumbs

1. Preheat oven to 325°F.
2. Steam or microwave broccoli until just barely soft, about 4 minutes; do not overcook.
3. Sauté onions and garlic in olive oil in a medium pan over medium-high heat until soft, about 3–4 minutes. Reduce heat to medium and add flour, stirring continuously to combine.
4. Add soy milk and vegetable broth and heat, stirring until thickened. Remove from heat and stir in nutritional yeast, margarine, nutmeg, mustard powder, and salt.
5. Combine sauce, broccoli, and cooked rice and transfer to a greased (with vegetable cooking spray) 9" square casserole or baking dish. Sprinkle top with bread crumbs.
6. Cover and bake for 25 minutes. Uncover and cook for another 10 minutes.

Per Serving
Calories: 485 | Fat: 11.0 grams | Sodium: 609 milligrams
Fiber: 7.0 grams | Carbohydrates: 79.4 grams
Net Carbohydrates: 72.4 grams | Sugar: 5.6 grams
Protein: 16.0 grams

Bulgur Wheat Tabbouleh Salad with Tomatoes

INGREDIENTS

Serves 4

1 ¼ cups vegetable broth
1 cup bulgur wheat
3 tablespoons olive oil
¼ cup lemon juice
1 teaspoon garlic powder
½ teaspoon salt
½ teaspoon black pepper
3 scallions, chopped
½ cup chopped fresh mint
½ cup chopped fresh parsley
1 (15-ounce) can chickpeas, drained and rinsed
3 large red ripe tomatoes, cored and diced

1. In a large bowl, pour broth over bulgur wheat. Cover and allow to sit for about 30 minutes until bulgur wheat is soft.
2. Toss bulgur wheat with olive oil, lemon juice, garlic powder, and salt, stirring well to coat. Combine with remaining ingredients, adding in tomatoes last.
3. Allow to chill for at least 1 hour before serving.

Per Serving
Calories: 341 | Fat: 11.6 grams | Sodium: 618 milligrams
Fiber: 11.3 grams | Carbohydrates: 51.0 grams
Net Carbohydrates: 39.7 grams | Sugar: 7.3 grams
Protein: 10.8 grams

....

LEFTOVER TABBOULEH SANDWICHES
Spread a slice of bread or a tortilla with some hummus, then layer leftover tabbouleh, sweet pickle relish, thinly sliced cucumbers, and some lettuce to make a quick sandwich or wrap for lunch.

....

Chapter 19

Sides: Salads and Vegetables

Edamame Salad

INGREDIENTS

Serves 4

2 cups frozen shelled edamame, thawed and drained

1 medium red bell pepper, seeded and diced

¾ cup frozen corn kernels, thawed

3 tablespoons chopped fresh cilantro

3 tablespoons olive oil

2 tablespoons red wine vinegar

1 teaspoon soy sauce

1 teaspoon chili powder

2 teaspoons lime juice

¼ teaspoon salt

⅛ teaspoon black pepper

1. In a large bowl, combine edamame, bell pepper, corn, and cilantro.
2. In a medium bowl, whisk together olive oil, vinegar, soy sauce, chili powder, and lime juice; combine with edamame. Add salt and black pepper.
3. Chill for at least 1 hour before serving.

Per Serving
Calories: 190 | Fat: 10.3 grams | Sodium: 246 milligrams
Fiber: 4.3 grams | Carbohydrates: 12.6 grams
Net Carbohydrates: 8.3 grams | Sugar: 4.5 grams
Protein: 7.5 grams

Spicy Sweet Cucumber Salad

INGREDIENTS

Serves 2

2 medium cucumbers, thinly sliced
¾ teaspoon salt
¼ cup rice wine vinegar
1 teaspoon sugar
1 teaspoon sesame oil
¼ teaspoon red pepper flakes
½ medium yellow onion, peeled and thinly sliced

1. In an ungreased 11" × 14" baking dish, spread cucumbers in a single layer; sprinkle with salt. Allow to sit at least 10 minutes.
2. Drain any excess water from cucumbers.
3. In a small bowl, whisk together rice wine vinegar, sugar, oil, and red pepper flakes.
4. Pour dressing over cucumbers; add onions and toss gently.
5. Allow to sit at least 10 minutes before serving to allow flavors to mingle.

Per Serving
Calories: 88 | Fat: 2.4 grams | Sodium: 748 milligrams
Fiber: 2.0 grams | Carbohydrates: 15.6 grams
Net Carbohydrates: 13.6 grams | Sugar: 8.3 grams
Protein: 2.3 grams

Lemon Cumin Potato Salad

INGREDIENTS

Serves 4

2 tablespoons olive oil
1 small yellow onion, peeled and diced
1½ teaspoons cumin
4 large cooked red potatoes, chopped
3 tablespoons lemon juice
2 teaspoons Dijon mustard
1 scallion, chopped
¼ teaspoon cayenne pepper
2 tablespoons chopped fresh cilantro

1. In a large skillet over medium heat, add olive oil. Once oil is warm, add onions and cook until soft, about 5 minutes.
2. Add cumin and potatoes; cook for 1 minute, stirring well to combine. Remove from heat.
3. In a small bowl, whisk together lemon juice and Dijon mustard; pour over potatoes, tossing gently to coat.
4. Add scallions, cayenne pepper, and cilantro; combine well.
5. Chill before serving.

Per Serving
Calories: 355 | Fat: 7.3 grams | Sodium: 94 milligrams
Fiber: 7.1 grams | Carbohydrates: 66.4 grams
Net Carbohydrates: 59.3 grams | Sugar: 4.6 grams
Protein: 8.1 grams

Kidney Bean and Chickpea Salad

INGREDIENTS

Serves 6

¼ cup olive oil
¼ cup red wine vinegar
½ teaspoon paprika
2 tablespoons lemon juice
1 (14-ounce) can chickpeas, drained and rinsed
1 (14-ounce) can kidney beans, drained and rinsed
½ cup sliced black olives
1 (8-ounce) can corn, drained
½ medium red onion, peeled and chopped
1 tablespoon chopped fresh parsley
½ teaspoon salt
¼ teaspoon black pepper

1. In a small bowl, whisk together olive oil, vinegar, paprika, and lemon juice.
2. In a large bowl, combine chickpeas, kidney beans, olives, corn, onions, and parsley. Pour dressing over bean mixture; toss well to combine.
3. Season with salt and pepper.
4. Chill for at least 1 hour before serving to allow flavors to mingle.

___

Per Serving
Calories: 250 | Fat: 11.6 grams | Sodium: 578 milligrams
Fiber: 7.5 grams | Carbohydrates: 28.8 grams
Net Carbohydrates: 21.3 grams | Sugar: 4.6 grams
Protein: 8.2 grams

Baked Sweet Potato Fries

INGREDIENTS

Serves 3

2 large sweet potatoes, sliced into fries
2 tablespoons olive oil
¼ teaspoon garlic powder
½ teaspoon paprika
½ teaspoon dark brown sugar
½ teaspoon chili powder
¼ teaspoon salt

1. Preheat oven to 400°F.
2. Spread sweet potato fries on a large ungreased baking sheet; drizzle with olive oil, tossing gently to coat.
3. In a small bowl, combine remaining ingredients. Sprinkle over potatoes; coat evenly and toss as needed.
4. Bake in oven for 10 minutes, turning once.

___

Per Serving
Calories: 159 | Fat: 8.9 grams | Sodium: 254 milligrams
Fiber: 2.9 grams | Carbohydrates: 18.8 grams
Net Carbohydrates: 15.9 grams | Sugar: 4.4 grams
Protein: 1.5 grams

Maple-Glazed Roasted Vegetables

INGREDIENTS

Serves 4

3 medium carrots, peeled and chopped

2 small parsnips, peeled and chopped

2 medium sweet potatoes, chopped

2 tablespoons olive oil

¼ teaspoon salt

⅛ teaspoon black pepper

⅓ cup maple syrup

2 tablespoons Dijon mustard

1 tablespoon balsamic vinegar

½ teaspoon hot sauce

1. Preheat oven to 400°F.
2. On a large ungreased baking sheet, spread out carrots, parsnips, and sweet potatoes.
3. Drizzle with olive oil and season with salt and pepper. Roast for 40 minutes, tossing once.
4. In a small bowl, whisk together syrup, mustard, vinegar, and hot sauce.
5. Transfer the roasted vegetables to a large bowl; toss well with maple mixture.

Per Serving
Calories: 239 | Fat: 7.5 grams | Sodium: 409 milligrams
Fiber: 4.5 grams | Carbohydrates: 40.9 grams
Net Carbohydrates: 36.4 grams | Sugar: 22.6 grams
Protein: 2.4 grams

Roasted Garlic Mashed Potatoes

INGREDIENTS

Serves 4

1 whole medium head garlic

2 tablespoons olive oil

6 medium russet potatoes, cooked and cut into small chunks

¼ cup vegan margarine

½ cup soy creamer

½ teaspoon salt

¼ teaspoon black pepper

1. Preheat oven to 400°F.
2. Remove outer layer of skin from garlic head. Drizzle with olive oil, wrap in aluminum foil, and place on a baking sheet. Roast in oven for 30 minutes.
3. Gently press garlic cloves out of skins; mash smooth with a fork.
4. Using a mixer or a potato masher, combine garlic with potatoes, margarine, and creamer until smooth.
5. Season with salt and pepper.

Per Serving
Calories: 564 | Fat: 11.7 grams | Sodium: 437 milligrams
Fiber: 10.1 grams | Carbohydrates: 99.7 grams
Net Carbohydrates: 89.6 grams | Sugar: 5.4 grams
Protein: 11.7 grams

Orange and Ginger Mixed-Vegetable Stir-Fry

INGREDIENTS

Serves 4

3 tablespoons orange juice
1 tablespoon apple cider vinegar
2 tablespoons soy sauce
2 tablespoons water
1 tablespoon maple syrup
1 teaspoon ground ginger
2 tablespoons olive oil
2 cloves garlic, minced
1 medium bunch broccoli, chopped
½ cup sliced white mushrooms
½ cup chopped snap peas
1 medium carrot, peeled and sliced
1 cup chopped bok choy

1. In a small bowl, whisk together orange juice, vinegar, soy sauce, water, maple syrup, and ginger.
2. Heat oil in a large skillet over high heat, add garlic, and cook for 1–2 minutes. Add vegetables. Allow to cook over high heat, stirring frequently, for 2–3 minutes until just starting to get tender.
3. Add sauce and reduce heat to medium; simmer, stirring frequently, for another 3–4 minutes until vegetables are cooked.

Per Serving
Calories: 154 | Fat: 6.8 grams | Sodium: 505 milligrams
Fiber: 5.5 grams | Carbohydrates: 19.8 grams
Net Carbohydrates: 14.3 grams | Sugar: 8.7 grams
Protein: 6.1 grams

Chapter 20

Soups and Stews

Black Bean and Butternut Squash Chili

INGREDIENTS

Serves 6

1 medium yellow onion,
    peeled and chopped
3 cloves garlic, minced
2 tablespoons olive oil
1 medium butternut squash,
    peeled, seeded, and
    chopped into chunks
2 (15-ounce) cans black beans,
    drained and rinsed
1 (28-ounce) can diced
    tomatoes, undrained
¾ cup vegetable broth
1 tablespoon chili powder
1 teaspoon cumin
¼ teaspoon cayenne pepper
½ teaspoon salt
2 tablespoons chopped fresh
    cilantro

1. In a large stockpot over high heat, sauté onions and garlic in oil until soft, about 4 minutes.
2. Reduce heat to medium and add remaining ingredients except cilantro.
3. Cover and simmer for 25 minutes.
4. Uncover and simmer another 5 minutes. Top with fresh cilantro just before serving.

Per Serving
Calories: 235 | Fat: 6.9 grams | Sodium: 1,152 milligrams
Fiber: 15.0 grams | Carbohydrates: 40.8 grams
Net Carbohydrates: 25.8 grams | Sugar: 9.7 grams
Protein: 8.8 grams

Easy Roasted Tomato Soup

INGREDIENTS

Serves 4

6 large red ripe tomatoes, cored
1 small yellow onion, peeled
4 cloves garlic
2 tablespoons olive oil
1¼ cups unsweetened soy milk
2 tablespoons chopped fresh basil
1½ teaspoons balsamic vinegar
¾ teaspoon salt
¼ teaspoon black pepper

1. Preheat oven to 425°F.
2. Slice tomatoes in half and cut onion into quarters. Place tomatoes, onion, and garlic on an ungreased baking sheet and drizzle with olive oil.
3. Roast in oven for 45 minutes to 1 hour.
4. Carefully transfer tomatoes, onion, and garlic to a blender, including any juices on the baking sheet. Add remaining ingredients; purée until almost smooth.
5. Reheat in a large pot over low heat for 1–2 minutes if needed.

Per Serving
Calories: 146 | Fat: 8.2 grams | Sodium: 478 milligrams
Fiber: 4.1 grams | Carbohydrates: 15.0 grams
Net Carbohydrates: 10.9 grams | Sugar: 8.6 grams
Protein: 5.0 grams

African Peanut and Greens Soup

INGREDIENTS

Serves 4

1 medium yellow onion, peeled and diced
3 medium red ripe tomatoes, cored and chopped
2 tablespoons olive oil
2 cups vegetable broth
1 cup coconut milk
⅓ cup peanut butter
1 (15-ounce) can chickpeas, drained and rinsed
½ teaspoon salt
1 teaspoon curry powder
1 teaspoon sugar
⅓ teaspoon red pepper flakes
12 ounces fresh spinach, stemmed

1. In a large pot over medium-high heat, sauté onions and tomatoes in olive oil until onions are soft, about 2–3 minutes.
2. Reduce heat to medium-low; add remaining ingredients except spinach. Stir well to combine.
3. Simmer on low heat uncovered, stirring occasionally, for 8–10 minutes.
4. Add spinach and allow to cook for another 1–2 minutes, just until spinach is wilted.
5. Remove from heat. Soup will thicken as it cools.

Per Serving
Calories: 455 | Fat: 30.7 grams | Sodium: 781 milligrams
Fiber: 9.7 grams | Carbohydrates: 31.5 grams
Net Carbohydrates: 21.8 grams | Sugar: 8.8 grams
Protein: 14.8 grams

Barley Vegetable Soup

INGREDIENTS

Serves 6

1 medium yellow onion, peeled and chopped

2 medium carrots, peeled and sliced

2 medium ribs celery, chopped

2 tablespoons olive oil

8 cups vegetable broth

1 cup barley, uncooked

1½ cups frozen mixed vegetables

1 (14-ounce) can diced tomatoes

½ teaspoon dried parsley

½ teaspoon dried thyme

2 bay leaves

½ teaspoon salt

¼ teaspoon black pepper

1. In a large stockpot over high heat, sauté onions, carrots, and celery in olive oil for 3–5 minutes, just until onions are almost soft.
2. Reduce heat to medium-low; add remaining ingredients except salt and pepper.
3. Bring to a simmer; cover and allow to cook for at least 45 minutes, stirring occasionally.
4. Remove cover; allow to cook for 10 more minutes.
5. Remove bay leaves; season with salt and pepper.

Per Serving
Calories: 245 | Fat: 4.9 grams | Sodium: 1,080 milligrams
Fiber: 10.9 grams | Carbohydrates: 44.8 grams
Net Carbohydrates: 33.9 grams | Sugar: 7.9 grams
Protein: 6.2 grams

White Bean and Orzo Minestrone

INGREDIENTS

Serves 6

3 cloves garlic, minced

1 medium yellow onion, peeled and chopped

2 ribs celery, chopped

2 tablespoons olive oil

5 cups vegetable broth

1 medium carrot, peeled and diced

1 cup chopped green beans

2 small red potatoes, chopped small

2 medium red ripe tomatoes, cored and chopped

1 (15-ounce) can cannellini beans, drained and rinsed

1 teaspoon dried basil

½ teaspoon dried oregano

¾ cup orzo

¾ teaspoon salt

⅓ teaspoon black pepper

1. In a large soup pot over high heat, cook garlic, onions, and celery in olive oil until just soft, about 3–4 minutes.
2. Add broth, carrot, green beans, potatoes, tomatoes, cannellini beans, basil, and oregano; bring to a simmer over medium heat. Cover and cook on medium-low heat for 20–25 minutes.
3. Add orzo; heat another 10 minutes, just until orzo is cooked. Season with salt and pepper.

Per Serving
Calories: 246 | Fat: 4.9 grams | Sodium: 879 milligrams
Fiber: 8.8 grams | Carbohydrates: 45.2 grams
Net Carbohydrates: 36.4 grams | Sugar: 5.1 grams
Protein: 8.5 grams

Potato and Leek Soup

INGREDIENTS

Serves 6

1 medium yellow onion, peeled and diced

2 cloves garlic, minced

2 tablespoons olive oil

6 cups vegetable broth

3 leeks, sliced

2 large Yukon Gold potatoes, peeled and chopped

2 bay leaves

1 cup unsweetened soy milk

2 tablespoons vegan margarine

¾ teaspoon salt

⅓ teaspoon black pepper

½ teaspoon sage

½ teaspoon thyme

2 tablespoons nutritional yeast

1. In a large pot over high heat, sauté onions and garlic in olive oil for 1–2 minutes, until onions are soft.
2. Lower heat to medium and add broth, leeks, potatoes, and bay leaves; bring to a slow simmer. Cook partially covered for 30 minutes until potatoes are soft.
3. Remove bay leaves. Working in batches as needed, purée soup in a blender until almost smooth, or desired consistency.
4. Return soup to pot, stir in remaining ingredients, and reheat as needed.

Per Serving
Calories: 173 | Fat: 6.8 grams | Sodium: 1,009 milligrams
Fiber: 3.4 grams | Carbohydrates: 23.9 grams
Net Carbohydrates: 20.5 grams | Sugar: 4.6 grams
Protein: 3.8 grams

NO YEAST? NO WORRIES!

If you don't have nutritional yeast at home, don't panic. This recipe will still be fantastic without it.

Chinese Hot and Sour Soup

INGREDIENTS

Serves 6

2 cups seitan, diced small

2 tablespoons vegetable oil

1½ teaspoons hot sauce

6 cups vegetable broth

½ medium head Napa cabbage, cored and shredded

¾ cup sliced shiitake mushrooms

1 (8-ounce) can bamboo shoots, drained

2 tablespoons soy sauce

2 tablespoons white vinegar

¾ teaspoon crushed red pepper flakes

¾ teaspoon salt

2 tablespoons cornstarch

¼ cup water

3 scallions, sliced

2 teaspoons sesame oil

1. In a medium pan, brown seitan in vegetable oil for 2–3 minutes. Reduce heat to low; add hot sauce, stirring well to coat. Cook over low heat for 1 more minute; remove from heat and set aside.
2. In a large stockpot, combine broth, cabbage, mushrooms, bamboo, soy sauce, vinegar, red pepper, and salt. Bring to a slow simmer over medium-high heat and cover. Simmer for at least 15 minutes.
3. In a small bowl, whisk together cornstarch and water; slowly stir into soup. Heat just until soup thickens, about 3–5 minutes.
4. Portion into serving bowls; top each serving with scallions and drizzle with sesame oil.

Per Serving
Calories: 200 | Fat: 5.9 grams | Sodium: 1,400 milligrams
Fiber: 4.6 grams | Carbohydrates: 18.8 grams
Net Carbohydrates: 14.2 grams | Sugar: 5.2 grams
Protein: 17.3 grams

Chapter 21

Snacks and Desserts

Eggplant Baba Ghanoush

INGREDIENTS

Yields 1½ Cups

2 medium eggplants
3 tablespoons olive oil, divided
2 tablespoons lemon juice
¼ cup tahini
3 cloves garlic, minced
½ teaspoon cumin
½ teaspoon chili powder
¼ teaspoon salt
1 tablespoon chopped fresh parsley

1. Preheat oven to 400°F.
2. Slice eggplants in half; prick several times with a fork.
3. Place on a greased (with vegetable cooking spray) baking sheet; drizzle with 1 tablespoon olive oil. Bake for about 30 minutes until soft. Allow to cool slightly.
4. Remove inner flesh; place in a medium bowl.
5. Using a large fork or potato masher, mash eggplant together with remaining ingredients until almost smooth.

Per 2 Tablespoons
Calories: 79 | Fat: 5.7 grams | Sodium: 57 milligrams
Fiber: 2.8 grams | Carbohydrates: 6.3 grams
Net Carbohydrates: 3.5 grams | Sugar: 2.8 grams
Protein: 1.7 grams

Hot Artichoke Spinach Dip

INGREDIENTS

Serves 8

1 (12-ounce) package frozen spinach, thawed
1 (14-ounce) can artichoke hearts, drained
¼ cup vegan margarine
¼ cup all-purpose flour
2 cups unsweetened soy milk
½ cup nutritional yeast
1 teaspoon garlic powder
1½ teaspoons onion powder
¼ teaspoon salt

1. Preheat oven to 350°F. Purée spinach and artichokes together until almost smooth; set aside.
2. In a medium saucepan, melt margarine over low heat. Slowly whisk in flour, 1 tablespoon at a time, stirring constantly to avoid lumps, until thick, about 1–3 minutes.
3. Remove from heat and add spinach and artichoke mixture; stir to combine. Add remaining ingredients.
4. Transfer to a greased (with vegetable cooking spray) ovenproof 3-cup casserole dish or bowl; bake for 20 minutes. Serve hot.

Per Serving
Calories: 110 | Fat: 4.3 grams | Sodium: 503 milligrams
Fiber: 4.0 grams | Carbohydrates: 10.9 grams
Net Carbohydrates: 6.9 grams | Sugar: 0.6 grams
Protein: 7.3 grams

Mango Citrus Salsa

INGREDIENTS

Yields 2 Cups

1 medium mango, peeled and chopped

2 medium tangerines, peeled and chopped

½ medium red bell pepper, seeded and chopped

½ medium red onion, peeled and minced

3 cloves garlic, minced

½ jalapeño pepper, minced

2 tablespoons lime juice

½ teaspoon salt

¼ teaspoon black pepper

3 tablespoons chopped fresh cilantro

1. Gently toss together all ingredients in a large bowl.
2. Allow to sit for at least 15 minutes before serving to allow flavors to mingle.

Per 2 Tablespoons
Calories: 22 | Fat: 0.1 grams | Sodium: 73 milligrams
Fiber: 0.7 grams | Carbohydrates: 5.6 grams
Net Carbohydrates: 4.9 grams | Sugar: 4.4 grams
Protein: 0.4 grams

Roasted Red Pepper Hummus

INGREDIENTS

Yields 1½ Cups

1 (15-ounce) can chickpeas, drained and rinsed

⅓ cup tahini

⅔ cup chopped roasted red peppers

3 tablespoons lemon juice

2 tablespoons olive oil

2 cloves garlic

½ teaspoon cumin

⅓ teaspoon salt

¼ teaspoon cayenne pepper

In a blender or food processor, process all ingredients until smooth, scraping sides down as needed.

Per 2 Tablespoons
Calories: 91 | Fat: 5.7 grams | Sodium: 223 milligrams
Fiber: 2.2 grams | Carbohydrates: 7.6 grams
Net Carbohydrates: 5.4 grams | Sugar: 1.0 grams
Protein: 2.9 grams

Steamed Avocado and Shiitake Pot Stickers

INGREDIENTS
Yields 15 Pot Stickers

1 medium avocado, peeled, pitted, and diced small
½ cup diced shiitake mushrooms
½ block (6 ounces) silken tofu, crumbled
1 clove garlic, minced
2 teaspoons balsamic vinegar
1 teaspoon soy sauce
15 vegan dumpling wrappers

1. In a small bowl, gently mash together all ingredients, except wrappers, until just mixed and crumbly.
2. Place about 1½ teaspoons of filling in middle of each wrapper. Fold in half and pinch closed, forming little pleats. You may want to dip your fingertips in water to help dumplings stay sealed, if needed.
3. To steam, carefully place a layer of dumplings in a steamer, making sure the dumplings don't touch. Place steamer above boiling water; allow to cook, covered, for 3–4 minutes.

Per Steamed Pot Sticker
Calories: 46 | Fat: 1.5 grams | Sodium: 71 milligrams
Fiber: 0.7 grams | Carbohydrates: 6.2 grams
Net Carbohydrates: 5.5 grams | Sugar: 0.3 grams
Protein: 1.6 grams

TO STEAM OR FRY...
If you prefer your dumplings fried, heat a thin layer of oil in a large skillet. Carefully add dumplings and cook for just 1 minute. Add about ½ cup water, cover, and cook for 3–4 minutes. In dumpling houses across East Asia, dumplings are served with a little bowl of freshly grated ginger, and diners create a simple dipping sauce from the various condiments on the table. To try it, pour some rice vinegar and a touch of soy sauce over a bit of ginger and add hot chili oil to taste.

Classic Chocolate Chip Cookies

INGREDIENTS

Yields about 2 Dozen Cookies

⅔ cup vegan margarine
⅔ cup granulated sugar
⅔ cup dark brown sugar
⅓ cup unsweetened applesauce
1½ teaspoons vanilla extract
Egg replacer for 2 eggs
2½ cups all-purpose flour
1 teaspoon baking soda
½ teaspoon baking powder
1 teaspoon salt
⅔ cup quick-cooking oats
1½ cups vegan chocolate chips

1. Preheat oven to 375°F.
2. In a large mixing bowl, cream together margarine and granulated sugar; mix in brown sugar, applesauce, vanilla, and egg replacer.
3. In a medium bowl, combine flour, baking soda, baking powder, and salt; combine with wet ingredients. Mix well.
4. Stir in oats and chocolate chips until just combined.
5. Drop by generous spoonfuls onto a parchment-lined baking sheet; bake for 10–12 minutes.

Per Cookie
Calories: 206 | Fat: 7.4 grams | Sodium: 199 milligrams
Fiber: 1.7 grams | Carbohydrates: 31.7 grams
Net Carbohydrates: 30.0 grams | Sugar: 18.0 grams
Protein: 2.3 grams

Coconut Rice Pudding

INGREDIENTS

Serves 4

1½ cups cooked white rice
1½ cups vanilla soy milk
1½ cups coconut milk
3 tablespoons brown rice syrup
2 tablespoons agave nectar
5 pitted dates, chopped
¼ teaspoon ground cinnamon
2 medium mangoes, peeled and chopped

1. Combine rice, soy milk, and coconut milk in a medium pan over low heat. Bring to a very low simmer for about 10 minutes until mixture starts to thicken.
2. Stir in brown rice syrup, agave nectar, and dates; heat for another 2–3 minutes.
3. Allow to cool slightly before serving to allow pudding to thicken slightly. Garnish with cinnamon and mangoes just before serving.

Per Serving
Calories: 484 | Fat: 17.8 grams | Sodium: 75 milligrams
Fiber: 4.1 grams | Carbohydrates: 73.5 grams
Net Carbohydrates: 69.4 grams | Sugar: 44.2 grams
Protein: 7.2 grams

No-Bake Cocoa Balls

INGREDIENTS

Serves 4

1 cup chopped pitted dates
1 cup walnuts
¼ cup cocoa powder
1 tablespoon peanut butter
¼ cup unsweetened coconut
   flakes

1. Cover dates in water; soak for about 10 minutes until softened. Drain.
2. In a food processor, process dates, nuts, cocoa powder, and peanut butter until combined and sticky.
3. Add coconut flakes; process until coarse.
4. Shape into balls; chill 1 hour on wax paper–lined plate.

Per Serving
Calories: 373 | Fat: 24.9 grams | Sodium: 3 milligrams
Fiber: 7.9 grams | Carbohydrates: 36.6 grams
Net Carbohydrates: 28.7 grams | Sugar: 24.4 grams
Protein: 7.9 grams

VARIATIONS
Roll these little balls in extra coconut flakes for a sweet presentation, or try using carob powder instead of cocoa—these alternate versions are just as satisfying. Don't have fresh dates on hand? Raisins may be substituted, but skip the soaking. Even with raisins, you really won't believe they're free of added sugar. Hint: If the mixture is too wet as you're forming the balls, add more nuts or coconut; add just a touch of water if the mixture is dry and crumbly.

Pumpkin Maple Pie

INGREDIENTS

Serves 8

1 (16-ounce) can pumpkin purée
½ cup maple syrup
1 (12-ounce) block silken tofu
¼ cup sugar
1½ teaspoons ground cinnamon
½ teaspoon ground ginger
½ teaspoon ground nutmeg
¼ teaspoon ground cloves
½ teaspoon salt
1 (9") prepared vegan pie crust

1. Preheat oven to 400°F.
2. In a food processor, process pumpkin, maple syrup, and tofu until smooth and creamy, about 1 minute.
3. Add sugar and spices, then pulse again; pour into pie crust.
4. Bake for about 1 hour; filling should be set and crust golden. Allow to cool before slicing and serving, as pie will set and firm as it cools.

Per Serving
Calories: 256 | Fat: 9.3 grams | Sodium: 255 milligrams
Fiber: 1.8 grams | Carbohydrates: 39.7 grams
Net Carbohydrates: 37.9 grams | Sugar: 23.0 grams
Protein: 4.5 grams

Sweetheart Raspberry Lemon Cupcakes

INGREDIENTS

Yields 12 Cupcakes

½ cup vegan margarine, softened
1 cup sugar
½ teaspoon vanilla extract
⅔ cup unsweetened soy milk
3 tablespoons lemon juice
Zest from 2 medium lemons
1¾ cups all-purpose flour
1½ teaspoons baking powder
½ teaspoon baking soda
¼ teaspoon salt
¾ cup diced fresh raspberries

1. Preheat oven to 350°F; grease with canola oil or line two cupcake tins.
2. In a large bowl, beat together margarine and sugar until light and fluffy, about 3 minutes.
3. Add vanilla, soy milk, lemon juice, and lemon zest.
4. In a medium bowl, sift together flour, baking powder, baking soda, and salt.
5. Combine flour mixture with wet ingredients until just mixed; do not overmix.
6. Gently fold in diced raspberries.
7. Fill cupcake compartments about ⅔ full with batter; bake immediately for 16–18 minutes until done (a toothpick inserted in middle will come out clean).

Per Frosted Cupcake
Calories: 315 | Fat: 9.1 grams | Sodium: 350 milligrams
Fiber: 1.3 grams | Carbohydrates: 55.5 grams
Net Carbohydrates: 54.2 grams | Sugar: 36.8 grams
Protein: 2.7 grams

....

RASPBERRY CREAM CHEESE FROSTING
Combine half of an 8-ounce container of vegan cream cheese with ¼ cup raspberry jam and ½ cup of softened vegan margarine. Beat until smooth, then add powdered sugar (about 2 cups—more if necessary) until a creamy frosting forms. This recipe will frost one batch of cupcakes. Pile it high and garnish your cupcakes with fresh strawberry slices or pink vegan candies.

....

Chocolate Mocha Ice Cream

INGREDIENTS

Serves 6

1 cup vegan chocolate chips
1 cup unsweetened soy milk
1 (12-ounce) block silken tofu
⅓ cup sugar
2 tablespoons instant coffee
2 teaspoons vanilla extract
¼ teaspoon salt

1. Using a double boiler, or over very low heat, melt chocolate chips until smooth and creamy, about 5 minutes. Allow to cool slightly.
2. In a food processor, blend together soy milk, tofu, sugar, coffee, vanilla, and salt until smooth, at least 2 minutes.
3. Add melted chocolate chips; process until smooth.
4. Transfer mixture to an ungreased 8" square freezer-proof baking or casserole dish; freeze.
5. Stir every 30 minutes until a smooth ice cream forms, about 4 hours. If mixture gets too firm, transfer to a blender, process until smooth, then return to freezer.

Per Serving
Calories: 312 | Fat: 15.4 grams | Sodium: 132 milligrams
Fiber: 2.9 grams | Carbohydrates: 35.4 grams
Net Carbohydrates: 32.5 grams | Sugar: 28.2 grams
Protein: 6.3 grams

Appendix A: Additional Resources

ABCs of Pregnancy—General Pregnancy Information

Reliable, comprehensive sources of pregnancy information and support.

Ask Dr. Sears

With Dr. Bill Sears and Martha Sears, RN

www.askdrsears.com

March of Dimes

National Office

1550 Crystal Dr., Suite 1300

Arlington, VA 22202

888-663-4637 (888-MODIMES)

www.marchofdimes.org

Verywell Family

"An Overview of Pregnancy"

With Robin Elise Weiss, PhD

www.verywellfamily.com/pregnancy-signs-and-symptoms-4157416

The Visible Embryo

A pictorial tour of embryonic and fetal development created with a grant from the National Institutes of Health (NIH).

www.visembryo.com

Childbirth Education

Find a childbirth educator or obtain more information on popular methods of childbirth. (See also "Professional Organizations.")

HypnoBirthing Institute
110-2 Sheep Davis Rd.
Pembroke, NH 03275
603-856-8792
603-856-8341
https://us.hypnobirthing.com

Lamaze International
2025 M St. NW
Suite 800
Washington, DC 20036-3309
202 367-1128
www.lamaze.org

Marvelous Multiples
www.marvelousmultiples.com

Waterbirth International
P.O. Box 812576
Boca Raton, FL 33481
954-821-9125
https://waterbirth.org

Complications in Pregnancy

Educational resources and support for complications in pregnancy.

American Diabetes Association
2451 Crystal Dr., Suite 900
Arlington, VA 22202
800-342-2383 (1-800-DIABETES)
www.diabetes.org/diabetes-basics/gestational

Preeclampsia Foundation
3840 West Eau Gallie Blvd., Suite 104
Melbourne, FL 32934
321-421-6957
800-665-9341
www.preeclampsia.org

Sidelines High-Risk Pregnancy Support
3167 Bern Dr.
Laguna Beach, CA 92651
612-492-1353
www.sidelines.org

Having a Healthy Pregnancy
Resources for prenatal health.

Motherisk
The Hospital for Sick Children
555 University Ave.
Toronto, Ontario, Canada M5G 1X8
Alcohol and Substance Use Helpline: 877-327-4636
Motherisk Helpline: 877-439-2744
www.motherisk.org

Infant Health and Development
Essentials for a healthy start in life.

Keep Kids Healthy
A Pediatrician's Guide to Your Child's Health and Safety
https://keepkidshealthy.com

KidsHealth
The Nemours Foundation
https://kidshealth.org

Zero to Three
1255 23rd St. NW, Suite 350
Washington, DC 20037
202-638-1144
800-899-4301
www.zerotothree.org

Maternal and Infant Nutrition and Food Safety

Breastfeeding facts, support, and nutrition assistance before and after pregnancy.

ChooseMyPlate.gov
USDA Center for Nutrition Policy and Promotion
3101 Park Center Dr.
Alexandria, VA 22302-1594
www.choosemyplate.gov

Food Safety for Moms to Be
Center for Food Safety and Applied Nutrition
US Food and Drug Administration
5001 Campus Dr.
College Park, MD 20740
888-723-3366 (1-888-SAFEFOOD)
www.fda.gov/food/resourcesforyou/healtheducators/ucm081785.htm

International Lactation Consultant Association
110 Horizon Dr., Suite 210
Raleigh, NC 27615
919-861-5577
888-452-2478
www.ilca.org/home

La Leche League International
110 Horizon Dr., Suite 210
Raleigh, NC 27615
919-459-2167
800-525-3243 (1-800-LALECHE)
www.llli.org

Women, Infants, and Children (WIC)
Food and Nutrition Service
United States Department of Agriculture
3101 Park Center Dr.
Alexandria, VA 22302
703-305-2062
www.fns.usda.gov/wic/women-infants-and-children-wic

Postpartum Health Issues

Learn more about common maternal health issues occurring after birth.

American Thyroid Association
6066 Leesburg Pike, Suite 550
Falls Church, VA 22041
www.thyroid.org

Postpartum Support International
6706 SW 54th Ave.
Portland, OR 97219
Office: 503-894-9453
Support Helpline: 800-944-4773
www.postpartum.net

Professional Organizations

Need a referral? These professional organizations can help. (See also "Maternal and Infant Nutrition and Food Safety.")

Academy of Nutrition and Dietetics
Find a Registered Dietitian Nutritionist
120 S. Riverside Plaza, Suite 2190
Chicago, IL 60606-6995
312-899-0040
800-877-1600
www.eatright.org

American Association of Birth Centers (AABC)
3123 Gottschall Rd.
Perkiomenville, PA 18074
215-234-8068
www.birthcenters.org

American College of Nurse-Midwives
8403 Colesville Rd., Suite 1550
Silver Spring, MD 20910
240-485-1800
www.midwife.org

American College of Obstetricians and Gynecologists (ACOG)
409 12th St. SW
Washington, DC 20024-2188
P.O. Box 70620
Washington, DC 20024-9998
202-638-5577
800-673-8444
www.acog.org

DONA International
35 E. Wacker Dr., Suite 850
Chicago, IL 60601-2106
888-788-3662 (888-788-DONA)
www.dona.org

The International Childbirth Education Association (ICEA)
110 Horizon Dr., Suite 210
Raleigh, NC 27615
919-674-4183
https://icea.org

National Society of Genetic Counselors (NSGC)
330 N. Wabash Ave., Suite 2000
Chicago, IL 60611
312-321-6834
www.nsgc.org

Special Issues

Special issues in pregnancy and beyond.

The Hygeia Foundation, Inc. and Institute for Perinatal Loss and Bereavement
264 Amity Rd.
Woodbridge, CT 06525
800-893-9198
www.drberman.org/hygeiafoundation

International Cesarean Awareness Network (ICAN)
2593 Orders Dr.
Morganton, NC 28655
800-686-4226 (800-686-ICAN)
www.ican-online.org

National Down Syndrome Society (NDSS)
8 E. 41st St., 8th Floor
New York, NY 10017
800-221-4602
www.ndss.org

National Organization on Fetal Alcohol Syndrome (NOFAS)
1200 Eton Ct. NW, 3rd Floor
Washington, DC 20007
800-666-6327 (800-66-NOFAS)
202-785-4585
www.nofas.org

Office on Women's Health
US Department of Health & Human Services
200 Independence Ave. SW, Room 712E
Washington, DC 20201
800-994-9662
www.womenshealth.gov

Spina Bifida Association (SBA)
1600 Wilson Blvd., Suite 800
Arlington, VA 22209
202-944-3285
800-621-3141
http://spinabifidaassociation.org

Twins or More
Resources for moms and dads of multiples. (See also "Childbirth Education.")

Multiples of America (National Organization of Mothers of Twins Clubs)
Executive Office
2000 Mallory Ln., Suite 130-600
Franklin, TN 37067-8231
www.multiplesofamerica.org

Vegans

Resources especially for vegans.

Position of the Academy of Nutrition and Dietetics: Vegetarian Diets
www.eatrightpro.org/-/media/eatrightpro-files/practice/
position-and-practice-papers/position-papers/
vegetarian-diet.ashx

HappyCow
www.happycow.net

North American Vegetarian Society (NAVS)
P.O. Box 72
Dolgeville, NY 13329
518-568-7970
https://navs-online.org

VeganEssentials
1701 Pearl St. #8
Waukesha, WI 53186
262-574-7761
866-888-3426
www.veganessentials.com

Vegetarian Nutrition Dietetic Practice Group
https://vegetariannutrition.net

The Vegetarian Resource Group (VRG)
P.O. Box 1463
Baltimore, MD 21203
410-366-8343
www.vrg.org

The VRG's Vegetarian Journal's Guide to Food Ingredients
www.vrg.org/ingredients/index.php

Appendix B: Birth Plan Checklist

Consider starting your birth plan with a short note both to your provider and to the nursing staff that will be caring for you during labor and delivery. Explain your general wishes for a healthy and safe delivery, for joint decision-making should medical interventions be required, and for open communication throughout the process. Read Chapter 14 to learn more about birth plans. Then use this checklist as a guide to assembling the basics.

1. Where will the birth take place?
   - Hospital
   - Birthing center
   - Home
   - Other: _____

   _____

   _____

2. Who will be there for labor support?
   - Partner
   - Doula
   - Friend
   - Family member

3. Will any room modifications or equipment be required to increase your comfort mentally and physically?
   - Objects from home (for example, pictures, blanket, pillow)
   - Lighting adjustments
   - Music
   - Video or photos of birth
   - Other: _____

   _____

   _____

4. Any special requests for labor prep procedures?
   - Forego enema
   - Self-administer the enema
   - Forego shaving
   - Shave self
   - Heparin lock instead of routine IV line
   - Other: _____

   _____

   _____

5. Eating and drinking during labor?
   - Want access to a light snack
   - Want access to water, sports drink, or other appropriate beverage
   - Want ice chips
   - Other: _____

   _____

   _____

6. Do you want pain medication?
   - Analgesic (for example, Stadol, Demerol, Nubain)
   - Epidural (If so, is timing an issue?)
   - Other: _____

   _____

   _____

7. What nonpharmaceutical pain-relief equipment might you want access to?
   - Hydrotherapy (shower, whirlpool)
   - Warm compresses
   - Birth ball
   - Other: _____

   _____

   _____

8. What interventions would you like to avoid unless deemed a medical necessity by your provider during labor? Specify your preferred alternatives.
   - Episiotomy
   - Forceps
   - Internal fetal monitoring
   - Pitocin (oxytocin)
   - Other: _____

   _____

   _____

9. What would you like your first face-to-face encounter with baby to be like?
   - Hold off on all nonessential treatment, evaluation, and tests for a specified time
   - If immediate tests and evaluation are necessary, you, your partner, or another support person will accompany baby
   - Want to nurse immediately following birth
   - Would like family members to meet baby immediately following birth
   - Other: _____

   _____

   _____

10. If a cesarean birth is required, what is important to you and your partner?
    - Type of anesthesia (general versus spinal block)
    - Having partner or another support person present
    - Spending time with baby immediately following procedure
    - Bonding with baby in the recovery room
    - Type of postoperative pain relief and nursing considerations
    - Other: _____

    _____

    _____

11. Do you have a preference for who cuts the cord and when the cut is performed?
    - Mom
    - Partner
    - Provider
    - Delay until cord stops pulsing
    - Cord blood will be banked; cut per banking guidelines
    - Cut at provider's discretion
    - Other: _____

    _____

    _____

12. What kind of postpartum care will you and baby have at the hospital?
    - Baby will room with mom
    - Baby will sleep in the nursery at night
    - Baby will breastfeed
    - Baby will bottle-feed (indicate formula baby should be given)
    - Baby will not be fed any supplemental formula and/or glucose water unless medically indicated
    - Baby will not be given a pacifier
    - Other: _____

    _____

    _____

13. Do you have specific considerations for after discharge?
    - Support and short-term care for siblings
    - Support if you've had a cesarean section
    - Maternity leave
    - Other: _____

    _____

    _____

Index